Don't Buy *That* Health Insurance:
Become an Educated Health Care Consumer

The Educated Health Insurance Consumer's Guide to
Reducing Health Care Costs

By

K. R. Woodfield

This edition published by
Dog Ear Publishing
4010 W. 86th Street, Ste H
Indianapolis, IN 46268

www.dogearpublishing.net

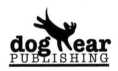

ISBN: 978-145751-532-3
This book is printed on acid-free paper.

Printed in the United States of America

Praise for
Don't Buy That *Health Insurance:*
Become an Educated Health Care Consumer

I think the book is extremely informative, especially for a small business owner. It explains a lot. There is a great need for some sort of consulting company to charge either small companies or individuals to help sort through medical billing and insurance purchase, and this is step toward understanding both.

—Joan Paoletta, Vice President, J. Cioffi Cargo Management

Your understanding and knowledge of the health insurance business played a large part in getting our insurance issued on a timely basis. I probably never met a sales person who worked so hard to talk me out of spending money!

-Nicholas A Lordi, Owner and President, Nalpro Business Solutions

Executive Summary

When I was younger, I was pretty sure I knew everything. My parents did not know nearly as much as I did. As I got older, I came to learn that they actually knew a lot more than I had originally given them credit for.

Since most of us use health care services and pay for at least some of our health care, too often we think we know all that we need to know.

For most people, the broker they use has become a trusted friend. After all, this is the person whom we trust to make sure that when the worst things happen in our lives, the financial floor doesn't fall out from under us as well.

Many of the brokers I have worked with tell the same story. They try to lead their clients to health insurance plans that will save the client money. However, the client does not always buy in on the broker's suggestions, for any number of reasons.

My goal is to give you the same information the broker has. *Before* you go out and buy or renew your health insurance, you need to read this book. When you have the same information that your broker has, the same knowledge and understanding of rates, you may realize that there are a lot of ways to save money on health insurance premiums.

I talk to a lot of people who way that they are afraid to make changes because they *feel* that they use a lot of services. They see the insurance company EOBs, explanations of benefits, and payments being made to various medical service providers and know that the policy that they have is good. It helps to mediate the costs of the goods and services that they use.

The next year, when premiums go up, the same people seem surprised. The great insurance that paid out several thousand dollars is now raising rates several thousand dollars! This makes sense, though, because the insurance companies are for profit business entities. They are not going to just give their money away. They want it back, the next year, and get it back through increased premiums.

How much is the entire health insurance premium?
What does your health insurance cover?
What are your predictable costs each month?

Understanding the answers to these questions is the key to reducing your health insurance premiums by 40–50 percent.

If your goal is to buy quality health insurance at an affordable price, this book can help you achieve your goal. The secret to achieving this objective is becoming better educated about the product you are buying. Educated health care consumers understand their own predictable costs and buy insurance that protects them against disaster. You don't insure predictable costs – you budget for them.

It's time to know what your parents know, know what your broker knows and know what the insurance companies know.

The free market is not at work until the consumer has price sensitivity. If you don't know how much the retail price of your prescription is, or how much your doctor charges for a sick visit, you have no price sensitivity. With prices hidden from view, we don't have a free market.

It's time to take control and take back your money.

Contents

Contents

Contents

Contents

Foreword

Becoming an Educated Health Insurance Consumer

How Much Does the Average Consumer Spend on Health Care?

While it is very difficult to determine how much the average consumer spends on health care, the US Department of Labor evaluates how we spend the consumer dollar each year. "The level of spending on healthcare continued to rise, from $2,853 in 2007 to $3,126 in 2009, largely due to the increase in the health insurance subcomponent."[1] That same Department of Labor report found that in 2009, health care accounted for 6.37 percent of the average consumer's dollar,[2] and health insurance accounted for 7.3 percent of the average employee's total compensation.[3] Based on Department of Labor statistics, we are paying a greater share of our income for our health insurance premiums than we are paying for our medical needs.

What is the average individual's annual risk of a hospital admission? The US Department of Health and Human Services, in its report as to the average cost of a hospital admission, points out the following risk statistics:

> In any year, most people do not need to be admitted to hospital—but those who do require hospital care face very high costs. Insurance is most economically valuable in the case of just such costly, but relatively rare and unexpected events. To put the figures above into context, the annual risk of a single hospitalization for an uninsured person is about two thirds as great as the annual risk that a driver

1

will be in an automobile crash (3% versus 4.59%), and about 10 times as great as the annual risk of a residential fire (3% versus 0.3%).[4]

The report further goes on to explain that "the average bill for a single hospitalization is about two and a half times the average economic loss (lost wages, medical care and other out of pocket expenditures) associated with an automobile crash ($22,200 versus $8,552)[5] and roughly equivalent to the average cost of property damage due to a residential fire ($22,200 versus $20,679)."[6] While these statistics have been normalized, the realization is quite clear: the average American is at a 3 percent risk of incurring a $22,000 medical bill.

A consulting company, Milliman, produced their annual research report on trends in health care in May 2011. Their report, *The Milliman Medical Index*, determines the average amount paid by a family of four for health insurance and health care. They do this by studying provider fees, benefits, and average health care use in all fifty states. Milliman also takes health insurance premiums, co-payments, deductibles, and coinsurance premium payments into consideration when defining health care costs. Milliman calls this an MMI cost.

The current 2011 study finds the MMI cost to insure a family of four is $19,393, an increase of $1,319, or 7.3 percent greater than it was in 2010.[7]

So let's review the statistics.

- Average American's risk of major accident or hospitalization: 3 percent
- Average American's annual out-of-pocket medical costs: 6.37 percent of his or her income
- Average American's annual health insurance premium: an incremental 7.3 percent of his or her income in addition to the annual out-of-pocket medical costs
- Total average American's annual health insurance + out-of-pocket costs: 14.3 percent of his or her income
- Average American family of four's annual health cost, including health insurance premiums: $19,393
- Average cost of a hospitalization: $22,200

Does it not seem ominous that we as a nation are paying almost $20,000 per year to insure a family of four against a 3 percent risk that they may incur a $22,000 hospital bill?

I believe we can reduce most people's health insurance premiums by 40–50 percent.

Profits were up on average 56 percent from 2008 to 2009 in the top five big providers, including WellPoint, United, Humana, UnitedHealth, and Cigna.[8] The first quarter of 2010 shows profits up again 31 percent over the same time period for 2009.[9]

An educated consumer can save money on his or her health insurance premiums. When you become an Educated Health Insurance Consumer (EHIC), you will be armed with insights to help you make logical and cost-effective choices about health insurance.

There are ways to save money on your health insurance premiums today. You simply need to know how and where to find them.

As a consumer in the current environment, we have very little information upon which to base our decisions. The following is a list of reforms that would make buying health insurance much easier:

1. Full health insurance plans in paper mailed to every consumer, outlining coverage and exclusions;
2. Universal common claim forms to reduce administrative waste;
3. Published contracted prices;
4. Annually published actuarial and risk tables;
5. A universal template of policy coverage and explanations that would result in transparency through standardization;
6. Optional participation in group health plans; and
7. Access to policy educators who will answer questions and explain coverage.

Until this is legislated, it is up to you to protect your family in a murky and seemingly predatory health insurance market.

You have an enormous amount to gain if you understand how the game is played. You also have a lot to lose financially if you don't stop paying into this money-churning system.

A Call to Action:
The Business Consumer and the Individual Consumer

Businesses and the officers who run them have significant buying power. Until now, they have primarily exercised that power through rate negotiation with the health insurance companies. Business owners and human resources professionals manage millions of dollars in premiums that insurance companies need to remain profitable. We need to get insurance companies competing for our business on our terms!

Annual rate increases abound as the health insurance industry tightens its grip on Congress.

No matter who you are, most people have trouble reading gibberish. Whether you run a company, work in human resources, or are simply protecting yourself or own family, we all have trouble wading through insurance policies.

Businesses have the right to demand that health insurance policies they are buying be presented with clarity. By launching an education-based initiative to understand health insurance, consumers will be better educated to understand the differences between policies and make better choices between options presented. Increased clarity will drive transparency.

Individual consumers need the opportunity and have the responsibility to read and understand the policies that they choose. Your health insurance plan should be presented in a consumer-friendly language that clearly outlines both the coverage and the exclusions in the policy.

The use of common examples in the body of the policy would help consumers considerably. They are helpful not only in understanding the costs associated with considering your options but also in understanding your coverage. Much like the consumer-friendly credit card legislation, clarity and uniformity will bring about knowledge and better decisions.

The large businesses and the individual consumer can work with industry watchdog groups to demand deliverables. The deliverables will be in paper format, educational, and easy to understand. The consumers will be educated and know how to maximize on their benefits while reducing out-of-pocket expenses.

The educated consumer has the power to facilitate and demand change.

Introduction

Why You Need to Read This Book

Do not go where the path may lead, go instead where there is
no path and leave a trail.
—Ralph Waldo Emerson

Americans *should* have access to affordable health insurance.
The national debate results from trying to work through an
obscure process that the health insurance companies have
intentionally kept murky.

Under the current system, you pay for many things that
you don't need. The insurance companies have created a system
that is complex and difficult to navigate. Many people *think* they
know what they are paying for with their health insurance.
Often, they do not know what they have until they use their
health insurance and find out what is *not* covered.

Health insurance providers do not disclose (even to
physicians) the rates they pay for services rendered. No one
knows how much is being paid for medical services until
payment is received. As a patient, you receive an Explanation of
Benefits (EOB) that shows only your responsibility to the
medical provider. It may also provide U&C (usual and
customary) fee information. You may think that is the rate the
provider is being compensated, but in many cases, it may not be
so. Too often this is just a number printed on a sheet of paper. It
may have no bearing at all to the amount the provider is paid.

In the absence of full disclosure, transparency and
useful information, insurance is purchased to calm a fear. The
fear is that if you seek medical attention, you might be charged
fees you cannot afford. Without data, you may be frightened
into buying health insurance that you neither need nor can
really afford.

Most people agree that health insurance is the best way
for individuals and families to protect themselves against
financial disaster brought on by extraordinary expenses at a

time of an accident or illness. The very high premiums you pay are divided between protection against disaster (an indemnity policy) and a "maintenance contract" (managed care). The maintenance contract reimburses you for day-to-day predictable and budgetable medical expenses.

Day-to-day expenses do not require insurance. Most current plans are maintenance contracts. In addition, the health insurance carriers are compensated an administrative fee for each and every payment they process. The health insurance company advocacy groups claim the fee is 3 percent of the average health care dollar. You will read later on that health insurance company audits put this fee anywhere from 11 to 40 percent of the average health care dollar.

This "managed care" component of your health insurance is the biggest factor driving up your premiums. Education is the key to understanding the real value of health insurance to each individual consumer.

Once you understand how the system works, you can lower your premiums. You will be empowered to make better choices and have more say in who provides your medical care. You can reduce your premiums without giving up the coverage you need.

As an educated consumer, you will know how to shop around and how to uncover hidden gaps in coverage.

Currently, there is a national debate about controlling health care costs. The large health insurance carriers point fingers at every moving part of the health care system, and there may well be a good reason for this. They are mindful, however, to take minimal responsibility for these increasing expenses themselves.

Education is the first step to moving from decision making based on fear to decision making based on transparency and facts. Only then can we understand how to reduce our health insurance premiums.

Issues and Solutions: Don't Gamble with Your Health Insurance

This book begins with a short history of health insurance and the birth of health benefits. The historical perspective lays the foundation for understanding where you can look to find savings.

Insurance has its own lingo. Each person may define words in his or her own mind differently. As a consumer of insurance, you should understand the language the health insurance providers use so that you may correctly interpret what you are reading. That is why there is a significant glossary at the end of this book.

 The Educated Health Insurance Consumers (EHICs) know that health insurance has a dictionary all its own. They learn how the insurers define words and read your plans knowing these definitions. EHICs do not fall prey to paying more for a plan because they imposed their understanding of a term over the definition used by the health insurance providers.

Chapter 1

You Are Not the Beneficiary of Your Health Insurance

Insurance is designed to indemnify (protect you against) a significant loss or financial disaster. It is not supposed to protect you against a seventy-dollar doctor's bill. One trip to the doctor is not a disaster.

All insurance works the same way. Think about the other types of insurance that you own. You may have homeowner's insurance. If something major happens to your house, you will be kept whole and be protected. Your homeowner's policy is there to put things right and get your home back to where it was before the disaster.

Consider your life insurance. Life insurance is designed to protect the people for whom you care, and to support them financially in the event that you no longer are able to provide for them. You designate the beneficiary; the people who get the check.

Car insurance is another place where you see the check and choose where it is paid. You are protecting your assets, your car, and your liability (the damage you may do to another). You are a part of the entire process when you have a collision repair done. You know how much each part costs up front. You know how much your deductible will be. You reaffirm your deductible every year when you sign up for the new policy. You might even manage your own risk of rate hikes. You might not report every ding and bump to the insurance company to protect your rates.

In every case but our American health care system, insurance *benefits*, *protects* and *pays* the policyholder or the policyholder's designees.

Who is the beneficiary of health insurance? And who is getting paid how much? As a health insurance agent, I ask this of people every day. Almost without fail, policyholders tell me that *they* benefit from having health insurance. This answer is correct, but it is only part of the complete answer.

"So," I ask them, "does that mean that you get a check from your health insurance provider when you go to the doctor?"

"Of course not," they reply. The checks go directly to the provider of the services, bypassing the consumer. You may never see the way the cogs move through the health care system.

 We don't see how much the provider thinks the charge should be.

 We don't know why the provider submitted the charge that we do see.

 We don't know how much is paid to the provider.

 We don't know how our co-pay fits into the equation.

We don't really understand how costs are getting out of control and why health care spending is becoming such a significant burden.

The check does not bypass you by accident—it is all part of a carefully constructed design.[1]

Insurance Fraud Launched "Coordinated Benefits"

Up until the 1970s, some people might have had more than one health insurance provider. Some opportunistic and creative people realized they could insure themselves with multiple health insurance policies. Then from one medical visit, they would file the same claim multiple times to multiple providers. They would receive several checks in the mail. After using one to pay the health care provider, they would pocket the others. This was profitable and it was also insurance fraud.

All types of insurance, health insurance included, are designed to keep you financially whole, not to make you rich. Because of the ease with which consumers could commit fraud, that system had to change.

The health insurance industry worked together to create a master system which they call "coordinating benefits." Insurance providers can see each other's claims. This avoids duplicity of payment from multiple providers for a particular claim. Consequently, the recipient (i.e., the beneficiary) of your health insurance dollar is not you. Instead, the cash benefit is paid to the medical service provider or claimant (i.e., the beneficiary) whose services were rendered.

This is the reason that you are not the beneficiary of your insurance payment. By not seeing the check, you have no idea how much is being paid to your medical services provider (i.e., the beneficiary). You are the beneficiary of the medical services or products rendered, but not the financial beneficiary of your policy. You no longer know how much you are paying for the services you receive. Only the insurance providers can see that information.

You also don't see the component parts of the various contracts the health insurance companies have signed with the health care providers. This is intentional.

The result is that the free market is stymied. You have no idea of the price you are paying to a provider to cover your day-to-day financially manageable medical expenses.

Likewise, we don't know how our policies are priced. Most of us don't know the cost of the indemnity portion of our policies. We don't know the cost of the managed care portion of our policies. We may not know how much we are paying for prescription coverage. We don't see how these components and other costs contribute to our premium cost.

In the absence of full disclosure of prices, the free market is stymied. To save money on health care, the consumer needs price sensitivity. Until we know relative prices, we are not sensitive to how and why they change.

Health Insurance Companies Consider Paying a Claim as a Loss of Income

Uncovering these contracted prices for services will give you new insight into the health insurance industry. Frequently blamed—and perhaps correctly so—it is not only the providers of the medical services that cause health insurance rates to increase.

You purchase health insurance to protect you from financial disaster. Health insurance companies are for-profit institutions and they need to maximize returns. You are both their source of income and their source of expense. You are the income because they collect your premiums and make a profit off of every single transaction that occurs in your health care. When they pay out a claim, it is an expense. This expense is called a Medical Loss Ratio (MLR).

Wendell Potter, the author of *Deadly Spin: An Insurance Company Insider Speaks Out on How Corporate PR Is Killing Health Care and Deceiving Americans*, explains how the health insurance companies use MLR.

 By jacking up premiums and shifting more and more cost to their policy holders, insurers are able to manipulate an obscure ratio that is especially important to their shareholders: MLR. It is telling that insurers consider the amount of money paid out in medical claims to be a loss. (Some companies now call it by other names, such as the "benefit ratio," which may sound more palatable.) When an insurer lowers its MLR, it is spending less on medical care and more on overhead …. If an insurer reports that its MLR was lower during the preceding quarter than the same quarter a year earlier, it means the company spent less on medical care—and therefore had more money left over to cover sales, marketing, underwriting, other administrative expenses and, most important, profits. This, in turn, pressures insurers to be vigilant in finding ways to cut their spending on medical care and this vigilance has paid off: Since 1993, the average MLR in America has dropped from 95 percent to around 80 percent.[2]

Health insurance companies offer contracts that offer "competitive" compensation to health care providers. They reduce losses (or expenses) this way. The insurance providers claim premiums are raised in reaction to increasing health care costs. Lower expenses and increased revenues improve shareholder return.

You can manage your own costs by first learning the fair market value of the goods and services you use. That is easy to say and fairly easy to do. In the workbook section of this book, I lay out a series of questions that you can ask your health care providers. This homework helps you to collect concrete information from which to base your decision.

The Answer to Why Your Health Insurance Rates Keep Increasing

Yes, there may be fraud in the health care system. There may be problems with billing and all the discussions currently being played out in the media may have validity. There is also another culprit contributing to rising health insurance rates. The total lack of transparency as to how health insurance companies operate gives question as to their contributions to this crisis. Consumers don't know how much they are charged for services or what services they are charged for. Providers don't know how they will be compensated. The industry is not regulated and there is no federal oversight.

Health insurance industry profits are soaring. Health insurance industry conditioning and fear mongering have consumers overpaying for insurance. A capitalist market is no longer at work.

EHICs know what their current medical costs are. They know how much money is a predictable outlay each month and each year. When you know predictable expenses, you reduce risk and reduce your need for coverage. When you compare your actual expenses against your health insurance premiums, you can determine which plan is the best for you.

Chapter 2

A Brief History of Health Insurance
(The Birth of Your Financial Burden)

In the absence of national health insurance, Americans have long depended on employer-sponsored insurance as the primary means of protection against the cost of illness.[1] Employers have shifted too much of the burden onto the working population, whose incomes are not growing rapidly enough for them to endure it.[2]

Every forty to fifty years, our health insurance system has changed as the times and the needs of the population have changed. Over the past century, each time the nation has been in the midst of a financial crisis, some sort of health care legislation has been created.

The Supreme Court ruled that insurance should be state based (as opposed to federally regulated) in 1869 in *Paul v. Virginia*. This was because the sale of insurance was determined to be "not a transaction of commerce." Since insurance was not deemed commerce, it was ruled as beyond the scope of federal legislation.[3,4]

That law was overturned seventy years later in a decision called *United States v. South-Eastern Underwriters Association*. Shortly thereafter, that decision was again overturned in the McCarran-Ferguson Act. The McCarran-Ferguson Act states that the regulation of the business of insurance by the state governments is in the public interest and that no federal law should try to regulate insurance.[5,6]

There have been attempts to restrict this law to benefit consumers, as recently as 2006. The failed National Insurance Act of 2006 was an attempt to pressure for federal reform of insurance regulation.[7]

Many people do not realize that each state governs how insurance is sold and issued to its citizens. This further clouds the learning environment, as laws vary from state to state. When people compare their experiences with health insurance, if they are talking to friends in another state, laws and knowledge may not lead to a better understanding. That is why consumers need to understand their own state's laws and how their insurance works for them.

In the Beginning, Health Insurance Was Not-for-Profit

Let's start at the birth of health benefits. In the beginning, there were "the Blues," Blue Cross and Blue Shield. They were not-for-profit organizations. During the Great Depression, a group of not-for-profit companies selling prepaid hospital insurance plans became known as Blue Cross. A second set of plans was created to cover physician services, and they were called Blue Shield.[8] Together, these plans were called "major medical" insurance. And they were good.

In the early 1900s, health insurance was more similar to the disability insurance of today. Health care improvements and hospital advances from the turn of the twentieth century brought on the socially desirable need to try to bring medical aid to those who needed it. Rather than buy health insurance as you know it today, people purchased protection against lost wages due to illness or serious injury. The premiums were not related to the costs of everyday medical care.[9] At a time when the average yearly salary was a little over $1,000, and a good family savings goal was $5 each week, a hospital bill of $140 could lead to financial ruin.[10] This was the birth of health insurance. It was designed to protect a family's savings from dilution by a catastrophic illness or accident.

Health Insurance as Compensation in Lieu of Wages

The introduction of employer-based benefits, particularly health insurance, came about during a window of American history when the country and the world were in the midst of a huge financial crisis: the Great Depression and World War II.

The Stabilization Act of 1942 was enacted by Congress to manage massive budgetary deficits caused by World War II. The law, designed to control inflation, limited wage increases but allowed employers to recruit, compensate, and reward their employees through a system of benefits. Those benefits would be paid by the employer on behalf of the employees, in lieu of increasing their incomes.

This is how it came to be that employers today are the primary purchasers of your health insurance. Originally, employers offered pension plans and life insurance as a way to sweeten the pot and attract or retain employees. As time went on, some very forward-thinking employers began to offer health insurance or a similar type of protection against unexpectedly large hospital bills.

After World War II, employers expanded insurance offerings to include both Blue Cross and Blue Shield benefits.[11]

Most Americans buy all of their own insurances, except for their health insurance. They purchase homeowner's and renter's insurance without any subsidies from their employers. Why then do they rely so heavily on their employers to pay a portion of life insurance, retirement savings plans, and health insurance?

Employers Get a Tax Advantage in Return for Offering Health Care Benefits

Another major turning point came as the result of the Internal Revenue Act of 1954 which made employer-sponsored employee health plans deductible business expenses. Offering health insurance became a tax advantage. Employers saw it as a benefit they could again offer in lieu of raising wages, with a simultaneous benefit of reducing their tax liability. By 1962, 25 percent of the workforce had employer-sponsored major medical insurance. With help from the HMO Act of 1973, 79 percent of all American employees were covered by some type of health insurance.[12]

The original intent of the HMO Act of 1973 was to encourage the creation and proliferation of nonprofit health insurance providers through federal grants and loans. In 1981, nearly 90 percent of all HMOs were nonprofits.[13]

In the early 1980s, Congress eliminated the federal aid intended to support the nonprofit operations of nearly all of the nation's HMOs. In response, many of these organizations converted into for-profit enterprises. By 1986, 59 percent of all HMOs operated on a for-profit basis.[14]

As a nation, we have come full circle. The last big financial crisis resulted in changes to health insurance in the late 1970s. The nation and the world are again in the midst of a huge financial crisis. So, the topic of health insurance and benefits is front page news again.

The Birth of Your Financial Burden: Catastrophic and Maintenance Coverage Combine

Insurance companies and politicians are like Oreo cookies: the cookies and cream work well together but they are not very good for you.

Clayton Christensen explains how health insurance plans evolved in his book *The Innovator's Prescription.*

> To differentiate themselves in the markets for talent and for insurance, employers and health plans in the 1960s next began to promote "comprehensive coverage," which included reimbursement for *day-to-day health care expenses.* The best employers offered the comprehensive plans—with the least amount of employee contribution—to attract and retain the best employees. Before long, two types of employer provided health care assistance—*true insurance against catastrophic illness and reimbursement of day-to-day health care expenses—had been combined into single-package health plans.* This unwittingly induces a pervasive sense of entitlement that today burdens employers who struggle to remain competitive in the global market for their products.[15]

For the past one hundred years, each time the nation has been in the midst of a financial crisis, Congress has stepped in to try to reduce the negative impact of health care on the economy. The last time Congress made significant changes to the health care playing field was forty years ago. Back then, the players were not-for-profit insurance companies. Today, the players on the field are different.

The players on the current field are for-profit health insurance providers. An expanded base of medical services providers have been added to the game. Confused consumers with a global sense of entitlement to health benefits are also crowding the field. Finally, the playing field itself has also changed as we grapple with new national health care legislation.

The worst government is the most moral.
—H. L. Mencken on Prohibition

Prohibition was a failed attempt at legislating morality. The current health care initiative includes another attempt at legislating ethics. The question at hand is, what if someone decides not to seek medical care because he doesn't want to or cannot afford to pay for it?

It is not my job to govern my neighbor's decisions on many fronts, and health care is among them. Congress can reduce the negative impact of health care and health insurance but there is debate as to how this should be done. Only by giving individuals fiscal accountability for their own health care decisions can you overcome this enormous conflagration.

The 1973 HMO legislation expanded employee access to health insurance benefits in two ways. While attempting to create a procompetition environment, it also created a medical cost containing system.[16] The HMO legislation was a way of compensating employees while offering employers a tax loophole.

This is a fundamental conflict. Health insurance should be a safety net to prevent financial disaster: Problems begin when it is used as a mechanism of tax-free compensation.

EHICs understand that they receive benefits *in lieu* of additional compensation. When you are asked to contribute to the cost of your benefits, it equates to paying your employer for the privilege of working. EHICs choose how they will be compensated by their employers, and want the choice as to how their compensation is distributed.

Improvements in the economy are often measured by consumer spending. Consumers will spend their income as they see fit and they can drive economic recovery. If insurance rate hikes absorb a significant portion of a consumer's annual income increases, then consumers have less money to spend in the open economy.

It's Hard to Care When You Are Blinded to the Cost

The first step to controlling costs involves knowing what the actual costs are that need to be controlled. After all, how can you save money if you do not know what you are spending?

You know how much you pay for your car insurance premium. You know what can happen that drives premiums up and what to adjust to bring your premiums down. Your homeowner's policy tells you which eventualities are covered and which are not covered. In fact, both policies are sent to you every year, and it is your responsibility to read them.

When your employer "owns" your coverage, your employer is the one who receives the full policy. If you are one of the lucky few who does not have to pay a portion of your health insurance premiums, then it is likely that you really don't care that your premiums are going up. You may not care about the endlessly touted "waste in the system." That apathy is another arrow in the health insurance companies' quiver. The health insurance companies are thriving in the current environment. They do not want the playing field changed.

I have three children. When employers pay a large chunk of the health insurance premium, there are times during a meeting with employees that I feel like I am talking to my children. Children don't care how much things cost. They have no money and they keep asking for things. People who don't pay for health insurance really don't worry much about how it impacts someone else's bottom line. The drawback is that those employees who don't have to pay may react childishly: they don't understand the cost, they don't need to understand the prices and they really don't care.

From the health industry perspective, employer-sponsored programs reduce policy cancellations. Employers usually keep their bills paid, and employees have restrictions about when they can make changes to their policies. This is a very good way to keep people protected, policies in force, and premiums paid.

Fewer employers are willing to absorb the entire cost of rising health care premiums. Employees growing out-of-pocket health care costs are an upward-spiraling problem. It has become common for employers to require employees to pay a portion of their health insurance premiums. This is obviously an unwelcome deduction from the employee's pay. It is often accompanied by increased medical co-pays at the point of service. Many employees feel as if they are getting hit twice for increased health insurance costs.

It is easier to care about these changing costs when they affect each one of us directly. We are still blind to how much is being paid for medical services but we are beginning to feel the negative impact of the escalating premiums on our personal budgets.

When an employer asks the employees to contribute to the cost of their health insurance premium, it is called *cost shifting*.

"Cost Shifting": ## You Pay for Both the Premium and the Benefit

"Cost shifting" has many meanings and many broad implications. For the purpose of educating the health care consumer, we will focus on shifting the cost of health care premiums and co-pays onto the consumer.

As we discussed earlier, health insurance benefits were historically offered to employees in lieu of increasing compensation. Employers are shifting these costs back to the employees as a means of reducing and managing business expenses. Since employers are no longer increasing your compensation package by way of increased benefits, it is reasonable that you might expect an increase in your compensation by way of wage increases. Because of the recession and slow recovery, employers can often neither increase wages nor absorb insurance premium rate hikes.

It is becoming an accepted practice to "cost shift" premium expenses while keeping salaries at the current rate. The result is that the employees' take-home salary goes down.

The pool of employees who have the majority of their policies paid by their employers is shrinking. The pool of employees who pay a portion of the premiums is growing. It is time to start caring about how much you are paying for everything.

Posting Insurance Policies Online is No Substitute for Getting and Reading Your Policy in Writing

An educated consumer needs to be given—and then read—his health insurance policy. This can be very difficult because the abbreviations and the language used are often unfamiliar. You may call the provider or your agent to ask for clarification but many just give up and hope it works when they need it.

Busy people may not always have time to chase down the location of the policy online. A healthy concern for the environment and "being green" means that many people are not given a paper copy of their insurance policies.

Today's environmentally friendly approach to business can also make understanding your health insurance policy difficult. In a book entitled *Paper to Digital: Documents in the Information Age*, the author, Ziming Liu, compared which documents are better read on hard paper and which documents are a good digital read.

Documents that are better understood when read on paper include lengthy, serious, complicated, in-depth, important items that may require note taking or rereading.[17]

Documents that are a preferred online read are casual, easy-to-understand, one-time reads of the most recent information and online documents save money as they cost less.[18]

Insurance companies usually post a summary of your policy online, which is the opposite of what Mr. Liu might recommend for such an important document.

Hiding behind a screen of making ecologically sound decisions, health insurance companies create obstacles to understanding and education by electronically communicating policy details.

If only the quote above referenced health insurance reform and not only credit card reform.

Transparency through Standardization

My clients often have trouble understanding the documents they receive. A universal template of policy coverage and explanations could easily alleviate this problem.

> With this new law, consumers will have the strong and reliable protections they deserve. We will continue to press for reform that is built on transparency, accountability, and mutual responsibility—values fundamental to the new foundation we seek to build for our economy.
>
> —President Obama on the Credit Card Accountability, Responsibility, and Disclosure Act

 EHICs demand a full copy of their health insurance policy be mailed to them each year in writing. They read through the policy and seek to understand their coverage. They call customer service when they need clarification on a term or a section of their specific policies.

Banks were mandated in the last few years to make their credit card statements and any statements bearing interest charges easy for the average American to understand.

Why has this courtesy not been extended to our health insurance policies? If the policy is written for the employer, then a consumer-friendly version of the policy for employees should be written and distributed to all of the employee policyholders each year. Instead of just highlighting what *is* covered, it is also important to know what *is not* covered. Owning a paper copy of your policy is another step in making you an educated consumer.

Education is Voluntary, but Participation is Mandatory

Making benefits meetings optional further discourages customer understanding. When employers have brokers come into the workplace to explain benefits to employees, it is often offered as a voluntary meeting. It has been my experience that employees define voluntary as "I don't have to go to that meeting."

Laws and the health insurance companies mandate that an employer guarantee 75 percent participation in health coverage. That means that if a company wants to offer this policy to its employees, 75 percent of its employees either must have this coverage or be covered by another health insurance policy through a family member.[19] As an employee, there is legislated pressure for you to buy into, or participate in, employer-sponsored health insurance.

After you are pressured into participating in your employer's health care plan, you are required to make a personal financial contribution toward the plan premium. The only place where you have any control is if you attend the education meeting. For too many busy employees at work, education and understanding are optional.

Your health insurance education should not be optional. Participation in your plan *should* be optional. After all, it is your money you are spending.

EHICs demand accountability from their health insurance providers. They want protection that is as easy to understand as it is to purchase. They want everyday language used in health insurance policies and they need time with a policy educator to be sure they understand that for which they are paying.

Not only should the education be mandatory, but the plans should be presented by a policy educator. We learn and comprehend much more when we see, speak, and hear information. The same learning techniques should be part of the health insurance benefits presentation.

A few years ago, the Health Insurance Association of America (HIAA, now called the AHIP, or America's Health Insurance Plans) looked at the language in health insurance plans. HIAA is a health insurance industry member trade group and association. Even their pro-industry evaluation pointed out "that while health plans and insurance regulators make every effort to ensure that insurance contracts are clear, understanding them does require a significant degree of effort on the part of the consumer."[20]

The marketing pieces created by the health insurance providers and provided by the agents are meant to enhance the attractive and more positive features of a plan. They rarely disclose all of the plan limitations. Most group health insurance members are poorly informed about the plan's rules and coverage limits until they receive a summary statement after the open enrollment period.[21]

Even then, the benefit booklets don't always fully reflect the contracts between the members' employers and the health insurers. Maria K. Todd, president and CEO of HealthPro Consulting Consortium, a private managed-care consulting firm in Aurora, Colorado, explained that the seeds of some of the most common claims problems are sown when employers purchase health insurance for their employees.

She explains how human resources people purchase health insurance. First, Todd gives to the health insurance brokers a list of desired attributes of a health plan. The broker returns to the employer with options and plans featuring those

27

requested benefits. The employer evaluates which plans offer the best combination of desired features for the best cost. After the employer selects an insurer, the broker hands the employer a contract to review and sign.[22]

"But the average human resources director really isn't aware he or she is being given a boilerplate contract that favors the health plan," Todd says. "They may not realize that every element of the plan is potentially negotiable, and that they could hammer out improvements for the plan members."[23]

Health insurance companies distribute tomes listing health care providers who participate in their plans. These books are both contact information resources and advertising materials. As advertising, the bigger the book, the more names listed, the more providers you feel will be within your reach when and if you should need them.

This book may be all you really know about your health insurance company. Without transparency, the health insurance companies negotiate contracts with pharmaceutical companies, test service providers, hospitals, and doctors. Health insurance companies claim that they are negotiating and contracting on your behalf. If it is all to our benefit, why is there so little transparency?

The answer might be because the health insurance companies answer to their shareholders and not to consumers.

Chapter 3

What's the Big Secret?

Unless someone like you cares a whole awful lot,
nothing is going to get better. It's not.
—Dr. Seuss, *The Lorax*

The prices that are charged in the insurance industry are referred to as "usual, customary, and reasonable", or UCRs. Health insurers tell us that they use UCRs to determine how much of a claim they will pay. They tell us that UCRs are supposedly the "going rate" health care providers in a specific geographic area charge for services.

As a consumer, you can't get a list of UCR prices. Even court orders have done little to force insurers to disclose UCR rates. Insurers claim this information is proprietary (or secret) business information. There have been literally dozens of class action lawsuits brought by states and legal groups trying to gain access to this UCR data to no avail.[1]

To understand how securely guarded health care cost information is, I want to share a story about myself and a blood test.

Having requested a test from my OB, I went to the local medical laboratory office and asked to have blood drawn.

"May I see your insurance card?" the gentleman asked.

"I am going to pay cash," I replied.

He looked a little frustrated and led me into his office. The medical lab employee could not look up the cost of the test on a laminated piece of paper kept handy for cash-paying customers because he did not see many cash-paying customers. Instead, he got on the speakerphone, called the main office, entered two different sets of passwords into the phone system, and finally made his way to a human. Having cleared himself as an employee, he asked the cost of the three tests my doctor had requested on the form.

"It will be $177," he said as he hung up the phone.

"My doctor added two extra tests—I just want my thyroid tested. How much is the thyroid test, and how much are the other two tests?" I replied. (I was not questioning my doctor's motives, I was just curious.)

"You only get the one price."

"No," I returned. "I want you to find out how much each test is in case I decide I don't want to have one of them." The poor man rolled his eyes, got back on the speakerphone, entered the two passwords, reached the same human, and had to explain that I was the same client and that I wanted to know the cost of each test. He was given the prices. One test was $123 and the other two tests were $27 each.

Now, as a cash-paying, educated consumer, I could go down the street to the next local lab and get a competitive price. So I did. My research stopped there because my doctor had filled out a form for that one particular laboratory and the next laboratory needed its own form. Since I did not have the right form, there was no way they were going to tell me how much anything cost.

Prices are so secret that not even the lab employees are allowed to know them.

 EHICs are bold and ask the cost of products and services *before* receiving said services. They are not embarrassed to learn how much they are being asked to spend of their hard-earned money *before* they commit to spending that money.

I was recently contacted with the following question:

Dear KW,   May 31, 2011
    I have a shocking (to me) little story about insurance bargaining, or what might more properly be called insurance extortion.
    Last week, my daughter took her mother to a neurologist for a brain test, as she is beginning to exhibit signs of forgetfulness. This led to MRI and MRA scans of the brain area. Afterward, the lab told her that the MRI was covered by insurance (she has Medicare and Blue Cross-Blue Shield) but not the MRA. They said the charge for this test was $1,500, payable on the spot by check or credit card. However, if she left the office without paying the full amount, the charge would then be $2,500!
    This seems to leave no room for negotiation, and so she paid the $1,500. I would likely have challenged the legality or at least the ethics of such high-handed tactics and would have established the cost before, not after, the procedure, which increases one's bargaining leverage. (Of course, I was not there, and the lab may well argue that $2,500 is the actual cost, and a $1,000 discount is offered for immediate payment, but that was not how they presented the bill.)
    Is this kind of cost manipulation commonplace with high-tech and expensive tests? It seems to combine intimidation with price extortion. Could anything have been done after the fact to bring down the cost to the patient?
    What are your thoughts?

In my reply, I offered two pieces of advice, albeit in hindsight. The first was to request a letter of medical necessity for the MRA from the physician who ordered it. The second was to shop around to the other area providers and inquire as to the costs and discounts of both tests to cash-paying patients.

In that letter, the patient had the financial resources to pay the funds up front. Those patients who would have to make several payments to cover the charges (the patients with clearly lesser financial resources) would be asked to pay more. This example shows the need for oversight and equity in the health insurance system.

Federal oversight could also provide a means of registering and handling disputes, and provide protection against price gouging.

No One is Policing the Profit-Oriented Health Insurance System

Very few of us know the costs of tests that are ordered by health care providers. You might be surprised to learn that a test such as a mammogram can range in price from $210 to $1,050.[2]

Health insurance companies have been given ample opportunity[3] to offer pricing transparency voluntarily, but have failed to do so. Information disclosure is always good for the public. When asked how they bill, only 2 percent of doctors voluntarily offer any information.[4] Just as the Securities Exchange Commission created financial transparency in the US securities markets, so too legislation is needed to establish transparency of the health insurance industry.[5]

Health care costs have risen 2.4 percentage points faster than the gross domestic product (GDP) since 1970.[6]

 EHICs embrace federal oversight of an industry that is responsible in 2009 for 17.6 percent of the gross domestic product (GDP), or $2.5 trillion. With CMS projections that health care spending may be as high as 20.3 percent of the GDP by 2018, EHICs support constructive legislation to prevent large-scale profit taking from an industry projected to spend $4.3 billion.

You *Must* Care and How You Can Effect Change

Who cares what it costs to receive medical care as long as insurance is paying, right? That is a pretty common mantra. You might want to care because these costs are passed to the policyholders in the way of increased premiums. You pay more, just like everyone else.

Premiums are costing more, and quality is going down. Quality health care providers deserve to be compensated properly for work done well. Too often, insurance companies offer rate schedules to providers on a "take it or leave it" basis. A lot of quality professionals have chosen to "leave it."

Under managed care, providers agree to a contract with a specific fee for services when they join a "network."[7] You may have a private physician who evaluates the fees and determines that there is not enough compensation in exchange for the value of the services being offered. That fee has to cover the cost of being in business, including rent, office staff salaries, various insurances, utilities, and so on. Providers generally have little power under managed care to negotiate fees for services. They are forced to accept the rates that are offered or risk losing their patient base.[8]

So, the first reason you may choose to care is that your favorite physician may choose to stop practicing medicine. This is the person upon whom you depend when things are going wrong in your medical world. That caregiver may not be there when you want him or her because the health insurance companies have made it too fiscally challenging to be in business.

The price to cash payers is another reason you may choose to care. I personally went from being a well-insured individual to a cash payer when my spouse passed away. Disaster can happen at any time and any one of us can end up a cash payer.

Managed care has created a type of "supplier-induced demand" that sets compensation for physicians' services. Physicians have very little discretion over the prices they can charge.[9] Cash payers cannot be expected to pick up the balance of the costs not borne by the health insurance industry. When contracted prices are reduced, physicians may work to offset their losses by charging more to their privately insured patients[10] and to their cash-paying patients. When the cash-paying patients can't pay, the cost falls to the taxpayer, so we end up paying again.

We have to get involved in overseeing payments if we want to control costs and reduce premiums. That is how health insurance companies make money—they charge high premiums and pay out significantly less than they take in.[11]

If you had the choice of taking the money that is spent on your premiums and putting that money back in your paycheck, you would want to know how much you were getting. Reducing premiums puts money back in your wallet.

 EHICs know they can effect change. EHICs can reduce costs by demanding copies of the managed care fee schedules of the policies they own.

The following statistics are alarming and disturbing:

- Eighty percent of Americans reported that they were dissatisfied with high national health care costs.[12]

- Over forty-five million Americans are uninsured—more than eight million of them are children.[13]

- Approximately 15.6 million adults are underinsured.[14]

- Since 2000, premiums for employer-sponsored health insurance have been rising four times faster than workers' earnings.[15]

- The average employee contribution to an employer-sponsored plan has increased more than 143 percent since 2000.[16]

- Average out-of-pocket costs for deductibles, co-payments for medications, and coinsurance for physicians and hospital visits have risen 115 percent since 2000.[17]

- As a share of GDP, US personal health care spending has more than doubled over the past three decades.[18]

- Total national health expenditures are expected to increase to $4 trillion by 2015, when they are projected to account for 20 percent of GDP.[19]

- Americans pay more, both as a share of GDP and on a per-capita basis, than citizens of other major industrialized nations.[20]

- The United States ranks far behind its international competitors in terms of health outcomes (e.g., longevity and infant mortality), despite spending significantly more on health care.[21]

- Almost half of all Americans report that they are very worried about having to pay more for their health care or health insurance.[22]

- Fifty percent of all bankruptcy filings were partly the result of medical expenses.[23]

- Every thirty seconds, someone in the United States files for bankruptcy in the aftermath of a serious health problem.[24]

- One-half of workers in low- and mid-range compensation jobs and one-quarter of workers in higher-compensation positions reported problems with medical bills, or were paying off accrued medical debt.[25]

- More than 25 percent of those surveyed in a study by the Access Project reported that they were unable to make rent or mortgage payments or that they suffered bad credit ratings because of medical debt.[26]

The system for delivering health care in the United States is under great stress and the pressures are mounting. If cost increases continue unabated and employers persist in their attempt to shift more and more of the burden onto the working population, the ranks of the uninsured will continue to expand, health outcomes will worsen, more people will be forced into bankruptcy, families will dissolve, and all of this will dampen economic activity in the rest of the economy.[27]

Chapter 4

When Did a Checkup Become a Financial Disaster?

The obscure we see eventually.
The completely obvious, it seems, takes longer.
—Edward R. Murrow

Health insurance has transformed from a design meant to indemnify a person against catastrophic loss to an entity that covers all of our routine health maintenance—something no other type of insurance is designed to do.

Indemnify Against Disaster with an Indemnity Policy

Several dictionaries define "indemnify" as "security or protection against damage or loss," or "compensation for a loss sustained." In other words, insurance should be designed to protect a person or family from *financial damage or loss.* Going to the doctor for routine examinations or minor injuries or illnesses are not disasters!

Administration, underwriting, marketing, and processing all of these policies are taken out of the premiums we pay to the health insurance company. These costs contribute to the "health care cost" pie.

A disproportionately large piece of pie is the managed care expense or coverage for day-to-day expenses. It is not designed to indemnify you against expenses incurred from a hospital stay due to a major illness or injury. The managed care percentage of our health insurance premiums covers routine maintenance. This might be vaccines, checkups, "wellness visits," annual physicals, or minor illnesses such as the flu or a sinus infection. The indemnity portion of the pie makes up the balance of the expenses.

> Throughout the health care reform debate of 2009 and 2010, top health insurance executives argued that total industry profits equal only one penny of every dollar spent in the US health care system. That was a big part of the industry's effort to make people think—erroneously—that insurers have little to do with rising health care premiums. But, even using their one-penny formula, which would mean the health insurance industry, collected $25 billion in profits in 2009 alone. At that rate, over a ten-year period that penny of profit could finance more than 25% of the $940 billion health care reform law.

> Health insurance company executives—including me [Wendell Potter] when I was spinning for the industry—have consistently asserted that premium hikes as high as 40 percent are necessary to cope with rising medical costs. They also like to complain that hospitals charge private insurers more to make up for lower Medicare rates. This all fits the industry's self-portrait of powerlessness in controlling medical costs despite the fact that, collectively, the large insurers have as much purchasing clout as Medicare.[1]

The Difference Between Maintenance "Managed Care" Contracts and Insurance "Indemnity" Policies

One buys a maintenance contract to manage high costs over a predictable time. An example to consider is the cost of heating your home during the winter. As oil gets more expensive, you can smooth out predictable outlays of cash for heating your home by breaking down the cost over several months and paying an equal amount each month. This is not insurance.

Insurance is sold to protect you against losses resulting from a specific risk. You buy furnace insurance to protect you and your family against a disaster with your furnace. You ensure that you will get help at any time, day or night, in the event of a heating emergency. You are protected against the cost to repair the furnace, potentially several thousand dollars, because it will be absorbed by the policy.

The difference between home heating oil and furnace insurance contracts and health insurance contracts is that you know the cost of oil and you can change distributors if you feel you can get a better deal elsewhere.

Just as you do not expect the government to negotiate your home heating bill or your furnace insurance contract, you do not need the government to negotiate your health insurance. If you budget accordingly, you can spread the cost of winter heating bills and furnace insurance over several months, with minimal risk of an unexpected expense. This is the theory behind the HMO. If you live in a warm climate, you might not need to do this. If you are otherwise healthy, you might not need an HMO.

The lack of transparency and the unwillingness of the health care industry to openly share costs muddies the decision-making waters considerably.

If you go to a walk-in clinic, some of which are now located in drugstores and even supermarkets, you will find costs posted for various procedures. They also will tell you in advance, step by step, how much the cost of the visit will be. If you are paying cash, the cost does not come as a surprise.

The staff of the clinic will file a claim with your health insurance provider. This means they will let your health insurance provider know that you sought medical care and that you had a financial outlay for which you would like to be reimbursed. If these walk-in clinics can post their costs, why can't other health care providers?

(EHICs) want health insurance indemnity policies that protect them against substantial loss, not against routine maintenance. They seek to buy from providers with very little administrative overhead costs.

If you are willing to "self insure" the deductible, your premiums may be reduced by as much as 40–50 percent.

Self insuring, in this case, means that you take on the responsibility for paying the costs that make up the deductible. If you incur a cost, you will be expected to pay the provider of the services for your expense. You assume the risk of the first few thousand dollars.

There are administrative expenses that are saved here as well. Research shows that claims processing as an administrative expense can cost you anywhere from 11–29 percent of the cost of your premium.[2] If you assume processing fees are about 20 percent of the deductible, then with a $2,000 deductible, your premiums will be reduced by around $2,000 + $400 in administrative fees, or a total of $2,400, for the contract year.

Even if you end up spending the first $2,000 on medical care of some sort, you still save the $400 in administrative fees.

"I Didn't See the Doctor at All Last Year: Why Should I Pay as Much as Someone Who Is at the Doctor's All the Time?"

If you only see doctors once a year for a physical, you are like 50 percent of the American population. The Kaiser Family Foundation estimates that one-half of the US population contributes to just over 3 percent of the cumulative national health care costs. One percent of the population (the very sickest) accounts for 21 percent of the health care costs and 10 percent (people with serious chronic, underlying conditions) account for 63 percent of the health care costs.[3]

As a nation, managed care—HMOs, PPOs, and POSs, or "maintenance contracts for our bodies"—is killing us financially. There is a portion of the population that benefits from a maintenance contract—those with underlying illnesses needing continual care, and those who are at a high risk to need more care more often.

The 10 percent of the population with ongoing health care needs accounting for 63 percent of the health care costs are the only ones who need this type of coverage. They use the medical system more, benefit from the services of their providers more often and therefore, should pay a greater amount. This is the group that contributes the least to the health insurance company's profitability and costs them the most in claims.

For the majority of us, we don't really need all this added protection but we are paying handsomely to have it. When we don't use these plans, the insurance companies grow rich.

Insurance companies will argue that insuring the less healthy in this way is a losing deal for them. They argue that they need the premiums from the healthy population to offset the losses sustained by the people who use their plans more often and more heavily.

Given their extraordinary profitability during the past few years, this is a weak position. Let the ill select the health care that meets their needs. Allow the healthy to benefit from plans that meet their needs—lower cost plans with better indemnity against disaster.

 EHICs buy the type of health care they need. If they are part of the 10 percent of the population that has underlying diseases that spend 63 percent of the health care budget, they should have managed care plans. Most healthy people today fall into the 50 percent category that incurs only 3 percent of the medical costs and, therefore, only need indemnity against disaster.

HMOs: The Monster That Ate Your Health Care

Health maintenance organizations (HMOs) were born in the 1970s as a way to improve people's lives. But over the years, HMOs, PPOs, and POSs have become the monster that ate health care.

Over the last forty years, we have become more enlightened and knowledgeable about our bodies and how to care for them. We have learned to eat better and about the benefits of exercising routinely. Our health risks are different today from what they were in the 1940s or in the 1970s. Our employment profiles are also different from what they were in the '70s. If you want to use benefits to attract and retain good employees, then the benefits we need from our employers must be different from what they were forty years ago.

Medicine itself has evolved a great deal in the past four decades. Our insurance must also evolve and not remain mired in outdated choices. We need health insurance that works with today's lifestyles and today's national economy.

Even though we all know about proper nutrition and exercise and the harmful effects of smoking, many of us choose to run our bodies into the ground. It's a free country and that is our right.

Just because some people have more medical needs than others—either because of choices they have made, bad luck in the genetic pool, or an accident or injury—doesn't mean that everyone in the country needs a one-size-fits-all medical insurance plan. The fifty-five-year-old man with high cholesterol may very well benefit from an HMO. The twenty-two-year-old healthy college graduate, who works out frequently, eats right, and has no underlying medical issues, should have an indemnity plan.

Free Market Economy Be Dammed; You Are Being Railroaded

As an insurance agent, I speak with people every day who want to change their health insurance because they feel they are paying too much. "Too much" is a broad term. Are their monthly premiums too high? Are their co-pays too high? (I agree that you are likely paying too much on both fronts.)

In a free-market economy, you know that having several providers of similar goods makes for a more competitive marketplace. Paradoxically, mystery pricing has resulted in the death of competitive pricing in the health care insurance marketplace.

Employers find themselves in a very difficult place. As Regina Herzlinger explains, "they [employers] find it difficult to reduce their role in the selection of health insurance because of the tax preference attached to employers' purchase; but employees who perceive that they are using somebody else's money do not exercise their normal shopping muscles when it comes to health care."[4]

She goes on to explain how employers look to their human resources professionals to control health care costs. Human resources professionals thought that sourcing their health insurance benefits through one provider would decrease costs by increasing the magnitude of the sale. In other words, one large group contract should save money due to volume pricing.[5]

> The results have been awful. In a bad imitation of Corporate Purchasing 101, they reduced the number of their suppliers and turned to a new breed of managed care vendors ... tough business people (e.g., the health insurance companies) who scrutinize every health care dollar, especially those aimed at the sick .... Corporate Purchasing 101 does not work in health care. U.S. health insurance programs were essentially created by health services providers who wanted assurance that they would get paid for their services. Consequently, a strong relationship existed between the providers and the insurers .... The middleman in health care—the insurer—has always had a lot to do with the doctors we could use.[6]

In other words, if you have a specific doctor you want to see, it is going to cost you more!

Why Can't You See the Doctors You Know and Want To See?

Despite rising premiums, consumers have also begrudgingly accepted ever-increasing co-pays. Where you might have paid ten-dollar co-pays for an MD visit twenty years ago, you may now pay fifty-dollar co-pays per visit. Most people don't know that a routine doctor visit might only be seventy-five or eighty dollars. So, when they visit a "participating" doctor and pay a fifty-dollar co-pay, they pay a mere twenty to thirty dollars less than the actual cost.

What are you paying those high premiums for?

Consumers often give up personal preferences when their policies change. Because their employers changed plans, the employees changed jobs, or through personal choice in an effort to save money, employees feel disenfranchised from their health care providers. You may feel you can no longer see the doctors who already know your medical history because those doctors don't accept the new health insurance plan.

Consumers are allowing an insurance company to dictate who will give them their medical care—one of the most important and personal choices that anyone can make.

 EHICs go to the doctors of their choosing. They understand that the cost of the visit may be about equal to their co-pay and are willing to pay a fraction more to be treated by the doctor of their choosing. The caregiver may in turn choose to accept a lower cash payment. The doctor saves administrative costs, and can pass the savings on to the patient.

Let's continue with our automobile example. Where do you take your car for its routine maintenance checkups—to have its oil changed, its air filter checked or changed, and other fluids topped off as needed? I'm betting that you drive it to the car care center that is closest and most convenient to where you live or work. You might choose to go to a care center based on a personal or professional friendship.

Would you drive an extra half hour to make sure that your car was serviced at the location your insurance company told you to go? Of course not! But as consumers of health care services, that is exactly what often happens. You go where you are told to go. You see the provider that you choose from those providers who have agreed to work with your plan.

Would you allow an outside entity, a national corporation, to tell you which bank you could use? Of course not! You would consider that an invasion of privacy. Then why do you allow your health insurance company to dictate your choice of doctor?

"Because the doctor will charge me more if I don't use health insurance," you might say.

According to the Georgia Public Policy Foundation, when patients pay cash at the time of service to the health care provider for routine medical care, they save the medical office a tremendous amount of paperwork. The less time spent on administrative and billing expenses, the less overhead there is and the medical office can pass that savings on to patients. As a result, cash-based medical offices charge patients less, earn more, and devote more attention to their patients.[7]

When asked, most doctors indicate that they can charge their cash-paying patients less. They pass on the savings from not submitting and waiting for payment from the claim.[8]

You may feel that you do not have a lot of say in your health care anymore if the plan is managed through your employer. You reluctantly change primary care providers because a faceless insurance company changed a plan, a doctor's office manager signed a contract, or an employer changed insurance agents. You feel helpless in a sea of changing decisions that affect your personal health care. It is dehumanizing and makes individuals feel like cogs in a machine.

The Educated Consumer Chooses the Doctor

The solution, of course, is to be a proactive and informed consumer. No one is stopping you from making any appointment with any doctor at any time. You may call up a provider and seek his or her opinion for a fee. You may go to a walk-in care provider and seek treatment. All they ask is that you pay them at the time of service.

Here is another way that health insurance companies manipulate you. Let's assume that you sought a medical opinion from a provider to whom you paid cash. The provider offers to "file as a courtesy." That means they will send a copy of your paid invoice to your health insurance provider. Upon receipt, the provider is supposed to credit your deductible with the value of that visit. The health insurance company might send you some reimbursement, or what they would have compensated the office for your visit.

Several mysteries unfold at this point. Let's assume your provider completed the form honestly and correctly. That "courtesy filing" has led you to expect a reply from your health insurance company. It might be that your payment was applied to your deductible.

It is hard to know how much your deductible is being reduced because many health insurance companies do not routinely send out confirmation of receipt of courtesy filings. You may need to follow up and specifically request confirmation of receipt and how much was applied to the deductible.

When you have a higher deductible, you expect to pay the provider for the visit. You worry less about how your managed care company will apply credit and you keep your receipts for your tax professional.

 EHICs go to the doctors of their choosing for routine medical care. For hospital care, they work with their insurers to find caregivers who will accept payment in full for very large expenses. EHICs pay a little more for caregivers they choose, and very little when big financial expenses are incurred.

Chapter 5

What the Health Insurance Companies Are Hiding: The Need for Transparency

Show me one who boasts continually of his "openness" and I will show you one who conceals much.
—Minna Thomas Antrim, *At the Sign of the Golden Calf*

The lack of transparency and federal oversight has resulted in health care costs rising 2.4 percentage points faster than the gross domestic product (GDP) since 1970.[1]

How much do medical services cost? Do health insurance providers run their own businesses as cost effectively as they are demanding all the providers run their businesses? These are very hard questions to answer.

Every time you add another layer of cost, administration and profit to any system, costs increase. This is why the insurance companies need to keep you blind to what is being paid to medical service and care providers, and to their own internal administrative costs.

Within the health insurance arena, there are two expense areas that need to be evaluated. The industry itself keeps blaming the providers of goods and services while facilitating payment of their services. The health insurance companies have an "inside track" because only they know the prices being paid. The health insurance companies need to be evaluated for their administrative inefficiencies as well.

How Much of Your Premium Goes to Administrative Overhead?

In 2009, Thomson Reuters published a document entitled *Where Can $700 Billion in Waste Be Cut Annually from the U.S. Healthcare System?*[2] They discussed the usual culprits, excessive hospital admissions, redundant testing, and how end-of-life care make up a lot of the excessive expenses.

Running policy and plan quotes for clients and comparing costs and benefits is a standard part of my day. I discuss deductibles and show how assuming the risk of higher deductibles can reduce premiums 40–50 percent. One reason is that the insurance company charges you to administer all those little claims.

If you have ever run a business, you know that the "cost of doing business" is a key cost-control variable. For the millions of Americans who have never run a business, the size of that cost is very difficult to fathom.

Each health insurance company offers hundreds of plans to the public. Not only are we blind to the costs, but we are also blind to the lack of uniformity in the billing process. The Thomson Reuters report observes that "in healthcare, the serious fragmentation of providers, the large number of payers and resulting disparate systems and procedures significantly add to provider and payer administrative costs."[3] It goes on to discuss how (health insurance companies offering multiple) health plans must support multiple redundant systems "for underwriting, claims administration, provider network contracting, and broker network management." The cost of doing business costs billions of dollars.

The administrative costs examined in the report are staggering. They occur both on the part of the insurance company and on the part of the hospital administration associated with invoicing and seeking payment from these multitiered, multipayer systems. The report references a 2005 paper by the Medical Group Management Association estimating that a simplified health care system could yield $300 billion in savings in administrative costs alone.[4] It also references PricewaterhouseCoopers' health industries research. PwC estimated that "[operational] waste [is] $126 to $315 billion per year, with waste in the claims processing alone at $21 to $210 billion."[5]

The next time you have to fight what you feel is a wrongly denied claim, think about how much you are being charged by the provider to talk to the people you need to speak with to correct the problem.

Hospital waste is often a topic of cost control discussions in health care. Often neglected costs include the administrative costs associated with hospitals' insurance receivables. "The average US hospital spends one quarter of its budget on billing and administration, nearly twice the average in Canada. American physicians spend nearly eight hours per week on paperwork and employ 1.66 clerical workers per doctor, far more than Canada."[6] As Wendell Potter recently wrote, "[the Thomson Reuters report] might make you wonder what value private insurers actually add to the American health care system."[7]

Other Than the Health Insurance Industry, Can You Name Any Other Industry When Invoices Are Submitted with No Idea of How Much Will Be Paid?

Freedom of the press is to the machinery of the state
what the safety valve is to the steam engine.
—Arthur Schopenhauer

In a society such as ours, where everything you do is labeled with a bar code and a price, it is absolutely amazing that most people have no idea how much they are paying to the medical professionals whose services they seek.

There is no other industry where costs are so difficult to uncover. If you go to the mechanic to have your car fixed, you see the hourly rate they charge posted in front of you before you agree to have the work done. If you agree to the price, you pay what is charged for the parts and the hourly labor before you leave. If you do not like their prices, you simply drive to another garage, get another estimate, and make your decision on which garage to use based on your due diligence.

Your accountant has a schedule of fees. Your lawyer has a schedule of fees. Your doctor also has a schedule of fees, but no one seems to know what they are.

If you are a cash-paying patient, you know exactly what prices are being charged by doctors for their services. These prices may not be readily available and they are never posted on a wall.

Unless you go to five doctors to treat one medical condition five different times and pay cash five different times, you will not know what the going rate may be for a specific visit. Since it is customary to seek treatment only for one problem with one provider, you do not discern how much another like-minded provider might charge for the same services. There is no platform for competition.

When we seek a second opinion, it is to see if a medical caregiver might reach a desired remedy in a similar or different manner. During that same interview, it is unlikely that you will ask how much that provider would charge to help you to achieve your desired outcome.

The concept of asking doctors what they charge or comparing prices from one doctor to the next seems fundamentally uncomfortable to many Americans. Books have been written asking how we can put a price on a human life and the value of excellent medical care.

Other for-profit entities, such as concierge medical services that promote their services solely to cash-paying patients, have figured out how to charge for their services. The drugstore chains and supermarkets also have figured out how to price their services.

At my local pharmacy, which also offers a minute clinic service, there is a table of conditions, services, and published prices. "[Consumers] ... are shifting their demand for health care away from expensive, conventional physician offices with limited hours to affordable and convenient retail clinics. Especially when consumers are spending their own out-of-pocket money for health care and they have a choice, they prefer market-driven, consumer-driven options like affordable, convenient retail clinics over conventional physician offices."[8]

Clearly, this business model has figured out how to tell you what their medical services are worth. What is precluding the insurance companies from sharing the same information? Why the need for obscurity and the fear of transparency?

 EHICs do not wait for insurance companies to answer their questions about costs. EHICs work together to develop a platform of data collected by individuals, designed to illuminate the actual costs of products and services used in the health care industry.

Without an Audit, the Data Provided by the Health Insurance Industry Must Be Assumed to Be Bogus

Statistics are used by baseball fans in much the same way that a drunk leans against a street lamp; it's there more for support than enlightenment.
—Vin Scully

In my graduate school statistics class, we were taught that numbers can be made to look like anything that anyone wants them to be. The classic example is as follows: "three out of four dentists who chew gum prefer a particular brand". There is more we don't know about the context of the question than we do know. Were there only a few dentists interviewed or were thousands of dentists surveyed? Do dentists have superior taste buds to the rest of us? In what scenario is that information relevant? Are you implying one gum causes less damage than others? Are you implying the gum sticks less to teeth? Were these dentists paid for their opinion? What value does their opinion really have?

We need the context within which any data is presented to determine the value of that data. Without context, data is not very useful information.

Insurance companies have an enormous collection of data from which to make actuarial tables. From these tables, they make choices and decisions about our health care which we, as consumers, know very little about.

A platform of data sharing on prices for medical services must be collected independently of any insurance company input. If consumers create a database of real-life information, we can begin to determine the actual market value of what most health caregivers charge for their goods and services. When the free-market system is allowed to work, most of us will not need to depend blindly on HMOs, PPOs, and POSs to manage our day-to-day medical costs. We will not buy health insurance policies made in decisions fear, but rather we will make buying decisions based on sound financial reason and consideration.

How Do Managed Care Companies Compensate Contracted Doctors?

In my research, I came across a doctor who made great efforts to explain how he came to charge the prices that he charges. William E. Jones, MD, of Austin, Texas, explains that the way he had to bill was based on his contractual agreements with his health management organizations:

> First, it is important to understand that no doctor these days expects to collect more than a fraction of what he (or she) bills to insurance; so in most cases it doesn't make any difference if he bills $100 or $1,000 because he knows the managed care company is only going to pay him $80 anyway.
>
> However, until the advent of managed health care, most patients paid their primary care doctor themselves. Family doctors were mindful of this, so they used to keep their fees at a level that seemed fair to both their patients and themselves.
>
> Nowadays even the most modest of fees by primary care doctors are being paid by third parties (managed care companies, Medicare, etc.), and not by patients themselves. As a result, doctors give little thought as to how high their billed charges may appear to their

patients. Knowing that compensation is often at "break even" or less, many doctors have been forced to employ any method available to obtain the maximum reimbursement they possibly can from each managed care plan.

One technique virtually every doctor now uses is to automatically raise the fee for ANY service if ANY insurance plan ever pays him at 100% of what he bills for that service. Why? Because it is the policy of every insurance plan to pay either 100% of a doctor's billed charge or their "Maximum Allowable Fee" for that service, whichever is LESS.

Consider how this works in the real world. If a doctor bills an insurance plan $75 for a service but the company's Maximum Allowable Fee for that service is actually $80, the company is going to pay him only the $75 he billed and never even tell him that they would have been willing to pay up to $80 for the service. The doctor has thus lost the extra $5 of potential income. That may not seem like much; but it adds up to a substantial amount of money over a year, especially since most primary care doctors these days are scrambling just to remain solvent.

Since the insurance companies refuse to reveal their Maximum Allowable fee schedule, the only way a doctor can determine the "best" fee to charge is to keep raising his fees until he discovers the point at which there is *no* company that will pay 100% of his fee.

Thus it has become the policy in almost every doctor's office to automatically raise the fee for any individual service any time ANY insurance company pays 100% of the billed charges; since that is the only way the doctor can discover what each company's "Maximum Allowable" is.

Dr. Jones calls this "fee creep" because it has resulted in fees billed by physicians creeping inexorably higher (often to absurd levels) as they were ratcheted steadily upward to match the amounts being paid by those few insurance plans whose "Maximum Allowables" were perhaps "overly generous" at some point in the past.

Every insurance company has sharply reduced its reimbursements over the past several years; yet a managed care doctor would clearly be foolish to reduce the amount billed to insurance lest he receive less reimbursement than he could from even that one isolated company that might be willing to pay a few dollars more.

Since managed care doctors know that their patients won't have to pay any more than their $10–15 co-pay anyway, they don't have any reason to care how high (sometimes preposterously high) they may have raised their fees.

As the managed care plans continue to grow ever more malignant, many family doctors would love to be able to drop off some (preferably all) of these plans and transition their practices back in the direction of simple fee-for-service (as they had done) but they are caught in a trap.

The problem for these doctors is that each of their managed care contracts stipulates that they must bill the exact same fees to a cash-paying patient that they bill to insurance. This means that doctors cannot legally bill a cash-paying patient one dime less than they bill to managed care companies for that same service. While the managed care companies deeply discount what they actually pay doctors, these doctors are precluded by their managed care contracts from offering the same discounts to their cash-paying patients.

Most Primary Care Physicians (Family Practitioners, Internists, and Pediatricians) are thus caught in a paradoxical situation because their over-inflated fee schedule scares off cash-paying patients. The doctor is prohibited from reducing his "cash-pay" fee schedule as long as he is bound by the terms of even one managed care contract!

EXAMPLE: Suppose a doctor ("Dr. Welby") thinks a fair fee for an office visit ought to be $55, but a few rare insurance plans have been paying up to $85 for the same visit. Dr. Welby knows that the majority of the managed care plans are going to pay only $47 for what he has determined ought to be a $55 office visit. Dr. Welby would be foolish if he didn't set his fee at the higher rate of $90 for that same visit he feels is fairly priced at $55 to guarantee that he'll be able to collect at least the maximum amount he can from any company that is willing to pay more. In that manner, he assures that for those plans where he could collect $85 he can make up for the losses on the $47 reimbursements.

The patient's co-pay is a portion of the financial reimbursement. If you have a $15 co-pay and the Maximum Fee is $47, Dr. Welby can expect to collect $32 from the insurance company and $15 from the patient which adds up to the allowable $47.[9]

Dr. Jones of Austin, Texas, now has a cash-only practice and has posted all his prices clearly. The good doctor's prices are listed below:

**William E. Jones,
Austin, Texas
Fee Schedule:**

<u>NAME</u>	<u>EXPLANATION</u>	<u>FEE</u>
Normal Office Visit	This is my *standard office visit charge* when I see an established patient for *one straightforward problem*, such as a respiratory infection, sprained ankle, a routine follow-up visit for hypertension, etc.	**$58**
Extended Office Visit	This is what I normally charge if we attend to 2–3 different problems at one time. For instance, if you come in with several unrelated problems that you ask me to address during the same visit. This charge would also apply if you have a single problem that requires extra time to evaluate properly and then discuss with you (such as a new pattern of worsening headaches).	**$78**
Complete History and Physical Exam (well *child*)	The following tests are *included in this fee*: • Vision Testing • Hearing Testing • Complete Blood Count • Urinalysis	**$135**
Complete History and Physical Exam (age 18–39)	The following tests are *included in this fee*: • Complete Blood Count • Blood Chemistry (diabetes, liver, etc.) • Cholesterol Test • Thyroid Test • Urinalysis	**$255**

Complete History and Physical Exam (age 40–64)	The following tests are *included in this fee*:	**$350**

- Complete Blood Count
- Blood Chemistry (diabetes, liver, etc.)
- Cholesterol Test
- Thyroid Test
- Urinalysis
- Stool Test for Blood (guaiac)
- Pap Smear (women)
- PSA (men)
- Electrocardiogram (ECG)
- Pulmonary Function (lungs)
- Vision Testing
- Glaucoma Testing
- Hearing Testing

CBC (Complete Blood Count)		**$23**
Urinalysis		**$22**
Urine Culture	Includes antibiotic sensitivity testing	**$45**
Cholesterol Test	Includes liver function testing at no extra charge	**$43**
Thyroid Test		**$45**
Strep Test		**$18**

How Do Health Insurance Companies Compensate Their Top Executives?

Senior executives in most every industry are well compensated for increasing revenue and stockholder value. The same holds true for the health insurance industry. In February 2010, the AMA published a report looking at mergers and acquisitions in the health care industry, entitled *AMA Study Shows Competition Disappearing in the Health Insurance Industry*. The report outlines how competition in the health insurance industry is disappearing. With more and more states offering products from only one or two providers, the largest providers have a near-monopoly control in each state.

Consolidating business has resulted in impressive control over the national markets. In 2009, twenty-four of the forty-three states reported in the new AMA report that the two largest insurers had a combined market share of 70 percent or more. That figure is up alarmingly from 2008, when only eighteen of forty-two states had two insurers with a combined market share of 70 percent or more. "The near total collapse of competitive and dynamic health insurance markets has not helped patients," said AMA president J. James Rohack, MD. "As demonstrated by proposed rate hikes in California and other states, health insurers have not shown greater efficiency and lower health care costs. Instead, patient premiums, deductibles and co-payments have soared without an increase in benefits in these increasingly consolidated markets."

"An absence of competition in health insurance markets is clearly not in the best economic interest of patients," said Dr. Rohack. "The AMA has urged the Department of Justice (DOJ) and state agencies to more aggressively enforce antitrust laws that prohibit harmful mergers." Compensation for the executive officers who have successfully guided their companies to this level of market penetration and control is staggering, as you can see in the following chart.

Annual Compensation of Health Insurance Company Executives (2006 and 2007 Figures)[10]

- Ronald A. Williams, Chair/CEO, Aetna, $23,045,834
- H. Edward Hanway, Chair/CEO, Cigna, $30.16 million
- David B. Snow Jr., Chair/CEO, Medco Health, $21.76 million
- Michael B. MCallister, CEO, Humana, $20.06 million
- Stephen J. Hemsley, CEO, UnitedHealth Group, $13,164,529
- Angela F. Braly, President/CEO, Wellpoint, $9,094,771
- Dale B. Wolf, CEO, Coventry Health Care, $20.86 million
- Jay M. Gellert, President/CEO, Health Net, $16.65 million

- William C. Van Faasen, Chairman, Blue Cross Blue Shield of Massachusetts, $3 million plus $16.4 million in retirement benefits
- Charlie Baker, President/CEO, Harvard Pilgrim Health Care, $1.5 million
- James Roosevelt Jr., CEO, Tufts Associated Health Plans, $1.3 million
- Cleve L. Killingsworth, President/CEO, Blue Cross Blue Shield of Massachusetts, $3.6 million
- Raymond McCaskey, CEO, Health Care Service (Blue Cross Blue Shield), $10.3 million
- Daniel P. McCartney, CEO, Healthcare Services Group, $1,061,513
- Daniel Loepp, CEO, Blue Cross Blue Shield of Michigan, $1,657,555
- Todd S. Farha, CEO, WellCare Health Plans, $5,270,825
- Michael F. Neidorff, CEO, Centene, $8,750,751

Transparency is like air. It's not important until you are not getting any.

Chapter 6

Health Insurance Is a Gamble: Wouldn't You Rather Be the Casino?

To relieve the pressure of your medical bills, I'm going to recommend that you go ahead and drain your savings account.
—Michael Maslin, *New Yorker*, 12/11/1995

I don't like to gamble because I always lose. Casinos thrive because the house has risk tables and figures for gamblers analogous to actuarial tables. The owners and managers of casinos can predict with relative accuracy how much money will be lost and won at different tables and machines. Like health insurance companies, they don't set themselves up for failure.

How Much Does the Average Consumer Spend on Health Care?

These statistics are important, so they bear repeating.
While it is very difficult to determine how much the average consumer spends on health care, the US Department of Labor evaluates the consumer dollar each year. "The level of spending on healthcare continued to rise, from $2,853 in 2007 to $3,126 in 2009, largely due to the increase in the health insurance subcomponent."[1] That same Department of Labor statistic found that in 2009, health care accounted for 6.37 percent of the average consumer's dollar[2] and health insurance accounted for 7.3 percent of the average employee's total compensation.[3] Based on Department of Labor statistics, we are

61

paying a greater share of our income for our health insurance premiums than we are paying for our medical care.

What is the average individual's annual risk of a hospital admission? The US Department of Health and Human Services, in its report as to the average cost of a hospital admission, points out the following risk statistics:

> In any year, most people do not need to be admitted to hospital—but those who do require hospital care face very high costs. Insurance is most economically valuable in the case of just such costly, but relatively rare and unexpected events. To put the figures above into context, the annual risk of a single hospitalization for an uninsured person is about two thirds as great as the annual risk that a driver will be in an automobile crash (3% versus 4.59%), and about 10 times as great as the annual risk of a residential fire (3% versus 0.3%).[4]

The report further goes on to explain that "the average bill for a single hospitalization is about two and a half times the average economic loss (lost wages, medical care, and other out-of-pocket expenditures) associated with an automobile crash ($22,200 versus $8,552)[5], and roughly equivalent to the average cost of property damage due to a residential fire ($22,200 versus $20,679)."[6] While these statistics have been normalized, the realization is quite clear: the average American is at a 3 percent risk of incurring a $22,000 medical bill.

A consulting company, Milliman, produced their annual research report on trends in health care in May 2011. Their report, *The Milliman Medical Index*, determines the average amount paid by a family of four for health insurance and health care. They do this by studying provider fees, benefits, and average health care use in all fifty states. Milliman also takes health insurance premiums, co-payments, deductibles, and coinsurance premium payments into consideration when defining health care costs. Milliman calls this an MMI cost.

The current 2011 study finds the MMI cost to insure a family of four is $19,393, an increase of $1,319, or 7.3 percent greater than it was in 2010.[7]

So let's review the statistics.

- Average American's risk of major accident or hospitalization: 3 percent
- Average American's annual out-of-pocket medical costs: 6.37 percent of his or her income
- Average American's annual health insurance premium: an incremental 7.3 percent of his or her income in addition to the annual out-of-pocket medical costs
- Total average American's annual health insurance + out-of-pocket-costs: 14.3 percent of his or her income
- Average American family of four's annual health cost, including health insurance premiums: $19,393
- Average cost of a hospitalization: $22,200

Does it not seem ominous that we as a nation are paying almost $20,000 per year to insure a family of four against a 3 percent risk that they may incur a $22,000 hospital bill?

With far more statistical knowledge than most of us, casinos and health insurance companies "stack the deck on their sides." They don't make bets they know they have a better chance of losing than winning.

From actuarial tables, the health insurance companies know the risks and the probabilities that people they insure at various stages of their lives will incur less cost than they pay into the system in premiums. Remember the 50 percent of the population that is incurring 3 percent of the annual costs? The health insurance companies know their ages, health statuses, and where they work.

Like most of the American population, we don't have tables to know our risk of incurring an excessive medical bill. We do not have actuarial tables upon which to base our insurance purchasing decisions. We just want to be safe in case we do have a disaster.

When I present policy options to the human resources person at a company, I explain that adding a high deductible or self insuring their employees for the first $1,200 or $2,400 is like taking the profit from the casino.

The "house," or the casino, is betting it will bring in more money in customer losses than it pays out in customer winnings. As the health insurance broker, I break out the math and show the customer how to protect employees against financial risk. Given the low likelihood that one company's employees will all spend the full deductible, the employer and the employee can come out ahead.

Deductibles: There Must Be a Reasonable Out-of-Pocket Risk, or It Isn't Insurance Anymore

Insurers have not limited the amount of the deductible and thus the employee's out-of-pocket risk. The federal government annually defines the risk components that define a qualified high-deductible plan. Less scrupulous providers have taken the high-deductible plan as an opportunity to shift costs even further onto the consumer. This illicit activity has burdened some consumers with crazy deductibles.

There has to be a reasonable out-of-pocket risk, or it really isn't insurance anymore. I have heard many employers cite examples of $5,000 individual deductibles and even $10,000 deductibles. In Maine, for example, "enrollees had policies with $15,000 individual deductibles and $30,000 family deductibles."[8] Obviously, these losses would be crushing to most households!

What Are the Affordable Alternatives to Going Naked?

I don't agree with the decision to be uninsured.

If the insurance companies were paying out more in health care costs than they were taking in premiums, they might have a reason to argue for hefty annual health insurance premium increases.

In the face of years of record health insurance industry profits, educated consumers have the right to demand accountability for the increasingly high premiums.

Health care reform is clearly needed. Discerning what changes and where changes need to be made is very difficult. Policy makers continue to lean on the propaganda offered up by the very industry in need of reform.

As an example of the misrepresentation of data, the White House blog printed a "reality check" on Oct 9, 2009:

This morning America's Health Insurance Plans (AHIP), the health insurance companies' lobbying operation, released a study it commissioned in an attempt to confuse the debate around health reform. Linda Douglass of the White House Health Reform Office didn't mince words in her reaction:

"It comes on the eve of a vote that will reduce the industry's profits," Douglass told TPMDC. "It is hard to take it seriously. The analysis completely ignores critical policies that will lower costs for those who have insurance, expand coverage and provide affordable health insurance options to millions of Americans who are priced out of today's health insurance market or are locked out by unfair insurance company practices."[9]

Faced with these types of deceptive practices, in the absence of federal oversight, consumers must ask questions to uncover this deceptive behavior.

Consumers also need access to actuarial tables and a platform to compare to collect data. This data must be unencumbered by insurance company PR departments and their impressive abilities to spin stories. Until then, there are ways that educated consumers can find good coverage.

 EHICs know that to save money, they have to do a little homework. The path of least resistance got us where we are today. It's time to do things differently.

Chapter 7

How Health Insurance Companies Use Fear to Manipulate Your Decision Making

If you receive your medical insurance through your employer, you may feel that your choices are limited. Many small businesses offer only one health insurance plan. Very large employers offer a smorgasbord of medical insurance choices for their employees. This too can be very frustrating.

The next time your company's open enrollment period comes up, take the time to sit down and really study each of the plans offered. The plan with the lowest co-pay is usually the plan with the highest premium. It requires a change of perspective, but you are better off with a policy you will only use as a result of an accident or major illness. You should look at the plan with the highest co-pay.

How Can the Average Person Know What Information Is Coming from Corporate Spin and What Information Is Real?

As soon as the insurance industry touts data that it makes a mere 3 percent in profits, you know you are to disregard this information.

Health Care for America Now is a grassroots coalition seeking health care reform at a time when Congress is being steamrolled by corporate special interest groups. In their May 2010 paper *Health Insurance Industry Profits Surge Again: Fewer Members, Skimpier Benefits, Lower Spending on Care Add up For Investors While Consumers Suffer*, they discuss in great detail the enormity of ongoing quarter-over-quarter financial profiteering by the health insurance industry.

Profits were up on average 56 percent from 2008 to 2009 in the top five big providers, including WellPoint, United, Humana, UnitedHealth, and Cigna.[1] The first quarter of 2010 showed profits up again 31 percent over the same time period for 2009.[2]

The 3 percent profit story holds no water but helpfully sheds light for the average consumer to know when a story is propaganda. If you read an article and the profits mentioned are 3 percent, you know you are reading something propagated by the health care spin system.

The Alphabet Soup of Health Insurance

Health care today is made up of many acronyms and groupings of letters that the consumers have been convinced have different values. The most common groups of letters are HMO, PPO, and POS.

The Health Maintenance Organization (HMO) was created as a way of consolidating many levels of care under one organizational roof. Physicians were connected either literally (by being in one building) or figuratively (by contracts). This group included all levels of care from primary care physicians through specialists and hospital care.

In an effort to control costs, the HMO forces you to go through a "gatekeeper" who sends you on to the next step of the medical journey. The gatekeeper is the physician who determines the type of specialist you should see. The physician must write a note to send you to the next doctor. That next doctor requires receipt of the note before he or she will examine you.

All of the doctors who are part of the HMO are called "participating." Doctors, hospitals, and ancillary services that agree to a contract are guaranteed a predictable flow of patients. Participating providers are "preferred" providers, or "in-network" providers. The customer is encouraged to seek care with them and is rewarded by paying a lower out-of-pocket co-pay.

When HMOs were first introduced in the 1970s, they were touted as an excellent way to control medical costs.

HMOs are a good choice for people or families with significant medical needs. They help you to budget medical expenses by spreading those costs evenly throughout the year.

The gatekeeper system gave control and financial incentives to the primary care physician. It was an effort to control the consumer's access to more expensive specialists. The introduction of a note from the gatekeeper was accompanied by seeking prior authorization, or preapproval, for your visits.

Many Americans found the level of control HMOs have given their primary care doctor to be stifling. The complaints and the strictures on seeing only in-network doctors soon began to make consumers chafe.

"Attitudes toward HMOs began to change for the worse, however, when the big for-profit insurers began to take over. These insurers knew that the more HMO members they had in a given market, the more leverage they would have over local doctors and hospitals. Not only could the insurers demand deep discounts from doctors once they acquired significant market share, but they could also influence—through their reimbursement policies and coverage guidelines—how the doctors practiced medicine."[3]

 EHICs are not confused by the subtleties of language. They look at the words "preferred provider" and "in network" and know that they mean the same thing. They look at the monthly premiums and out-of-pocket costs and know that more coverage for a lower premium is a better choice than higher premiums for less coverage and some flexibility.

Feeling restricted, consumers demanded more choice. This gave rise to the PPO and POS, more costly alternatives to the HMO. Willing to pay a bit more for more flexibility, many consumers believe that PPOs and POSs are better policies than HMOs. They are often nicknamed "high" plans where HMOs are called "low" plans.

A Preferred Provider Organization (PPO) allows patients to see physicians who are outside of the "in network" (or "out of network") in exchange for paying a greater share of the cost associated with those hospitals and doctors. PPO providers are considered more high-end because they are "preferred." "Preferred" seems to have fewer of the negative connotations left behind in our memories by in-network gatekeepers. The premiums and co-pays are generally higher than the HMO premiums and co-pays. Logically, more doctors sign on to these plans because they are reimbursed at a higher rate than the HMOs. If more doctors have agreed to the reimbursement rate, the plans also may be called "richer."

The Point of Service (POS) version of HMOs provides plan members with partial coverage for certain services they get outside the managed care plan network of providers. It is a middle ground between a PPO and an HMO.

The trend to join PPOs and POSs caught on like wildfire. By 2006, 60 percent of people covered by employer-based insurance had PPOs, up from 18 percent a decade earlier in 1996. During those years, the percent of consumers enrolled in HMOs dropped from 31 percent to 20 percent.[4]

This trend goes against the common wisdom of wanting good value for your dollar. The consumers who belong to HMOs generally pay a lower premium, have lower co-pays, and have lower out-of-pocket costs overall. The consumers who belong to PPOs pay a higher premium and pay higher out-of-pocket expenses.

No doctor I have met over the past twenty years would change the diagnosis of your illness based on your payment schedule. They prefer to be paid a higher rate for their services and so they favor any agreement that compensates them better than another.

Using Language Against You

The letters HMO now have a negative connotation, and PPO or POS have a more highbrow and positive reputation. Remember, HMOs are usually the low plan and the PPO/POS are the high plans. "High" means it costs more, and it implies better things.

Each plan says the same thing—the subtlety lies in the choice of wording. What is fundamentally different about the phrases "in network" and "preferred provider"? "In network" sounds utilitarian, and "preferred provider" sounds more upper crust. Regardless, the insurance companies still drive you to see the providers who have agreed to their contracts.

The irony here is that you pay more to the insurance company in premiums and more to the health care provider in co-pays when you have a PPO or a POS. If you are part of the 50 percent of the population who incurs 3 percent of the costs, you may be oversubscribing to benefits.

Thus, HMOs cost the consumer less, but they are bad; PPOs and POSs cost the consumer more, and they are good. Insurance companies collect more in premiums and pay out less in benefits for PPOs and POSs, so they are very good for their bottom line.

Lower premiums, less out-of-pocket: when did that become a bad idea?

What to Do When Your Doctor Does Not Accept Your Plan

The following scenario may sound familiar to you. A doctor you have gone to for many years no longer participates in your plan. What do you do? I know it seems counterintuitive when you are paying for health insurance for which you expect universal coverage, but I suggest you *go to the doctor you like and pay for the visit.*

Practicing what I preach, I have done just this. I see my gynecologist once a year for a checkup. She does not participate in my new insurance plan. She charges me $150 for a visit. I am happy to pay that. If I had changed my HMO to a PPO that my gynecologist participates in, the up charge would have been $300 per month. That means my yearly cost to see my gynecologist one time would have been $3,600. I am saving money by paying cash to see the doctor that I want.

Those doctors who don't participate also have a hand in driving you to choose a more expensive plan. Most people have no idea how much it costs to go to the doctor for an annual exam.

71

EHICs ask what a doctor will charge for a visit if they do not choose to use their insurance plan. Armed with this kind of knowledge, you can make cost-effective and savvy decisions about personal physicians, and not choose a more expensive plan because a specific doctor is on it.

Not surprisingly, the insurance companies have done their very best to keep the cost of a single visit to a doctor a complete secret. We hear a lot about waste and about how doctors are overcharging. We are confused with terms like "usual" and "customary." In general, the consumer has no reliable facts upon which to make an educated decision.

Downgrade to an HMO: When Did Paying Less for Better Coverage Become a Downgrade?

Nothing irritated me more than hearing from a client preparing to have cataract surgery that he was annoyed by his deductible.

"You don't have a deductible," I told him. He is on a fixed income, is over fifty-five, and was a candidate for a number of health problems. For him, an HMO was an excellent choice. I had signed him up for the HMO only a few months previously.

He had received a letter, he explained, and had been upgraded to a PPO.

"You were *upgraded?* How much more is that costing each month?" I asked, somewhat confused. It was an increase of over $250 per month with a $2,500 deductible. The plan I had signed him up for had $50 outpatient co-pay (cataracts were this type of surgery) and no deductible. He also had to pay another 30 percent of the surgery costs (up to $10,000)!

I called the provider, and they explained that my client had received a letter offering to upgrade him the next month. His lack of response to the offer and subsequent payment of the new premium was an implied agreement that he had accepted the upgrade.

"Why didn't you call me when you got this upgrade letter? Did it not occur to you that I had intentionally *not* signed you up for the PPO?" I asked. His answer was that he figured that I had made a mistake by not signing him up for the more costly service. He was pleased they thought him a good risk and that the provider would "upgrade" him. The higher premium was simply the cost to be paid for the upgrade.

I asked the provider how to put him back on the HMO. "No problem," the provider's customer service agent helpfully replied. "You just need to request to be *downgraded* to the HMO." Same MD, same hospital, same surgery, and it is a downgrade to pay $50 instead of $2,500 plus 30 percent of the costs over $2,500? Only the insurance company can call that a downgrade!

 EHICs do not allow the health insurance industries' use of language to cost them more money. They make fiscally prudent decisions based on the facts, and not on the sociological value assigned to words.

The insurance manipulated the way in which the HMO is perceived. While "upgrading" and up charging happened automatically, the company made him request, in writing, to be downgraded to an HMO to lower his premium. So, I spent an hour reviewing the facts with my client, making sure that he understood the value of the change.

This insurance company used the word "downgrade" to repel the client from choosing a plan that saved him thousands of dollars. They did not use a neutral or more comforting word like "switch" or "change" or "exchange" or "modify" to give the consumer confidence in this decision. They were using English against him.

And then it happened again!

Another client and friend needed a new wheelchair. She explained to me that she was looking forward to getting her new wheelchair. Before the policy had been written, I had made several calls to ensure her new policy would cover the chair. We had also researched the in-network retail providers of her next wheelchair. When I ran into her, she was upset because it seems she had a $2,500 deductible on the new wheelchair.

Once again, there was a deductible on a client's policy that I had signed up for an HMO with no deductible. I asked her if she had received a letter offering to upgrade her to the PPO.

"Yes, how did you know?" she asked. I sat down and spent another hour explaining the problem and the process. Yes, she understood that the monthly rate was higher for her PPO "upgrade." It hadn't bothered her to pay more each month until she needed to get the wheelchair.

"I made sure you were on the plan where a new chair would be provided for only twenty-five dollars. Do not buy that chair until we switch you back," I implored of her. When I explained she would have to use the word "downgrade" in a letter, I saw her wince and begin to worry about her plan. She had to think about it and said she would get back to me.

 (EHICs) know the phone number for the customer service department at their health insurance provider. They feel very comfortable picking up the phone and asking questions until they have a satisfactory answer. EHICs ask questions and behave like "squeaky wheels" until they get the desired result.

Who has to think about spending $2,500 to get the same wheelchair that you could get for $25? The word "downgrade" really unraveled her.

Had she not been a good friend, she might not have trusted me enough to "downgrade" her policy. Finally, through a lot of support and hand-holding—and several phone calls and e-mails to her health insurance company—she did make the request and is now happily cruising in her new ride.

Getting people the right product at the right price and defending them against the predatory behavior of an insurance provider takes a lot of time and patience. Not everyone knows that they can fight for what they want.

Chapter 8

Insurance Agents: Your Ally or Your Enemy—Your Choice

Throughout the history of commercial life nobody has ever quite liked the commission man. His function is too vague, his presence always seems one too many, his profit looks too easy, and even when you admit that he has a necessary function, you feel that this function is, as it were, a personification of something that in an ethical society would not need to exist. If people could deal with one another honestly, they would not need agents.
—Raymond Chandler

There is a difference between being a broker and being an agent. When a broker represents a specific insurance company, he or she acts as an "agent" of that insurance company. To become an agent, you apply for an appointment allowing you to represent that company.

Insurance salespeople are paid by way of commissions. Most insurance professionals can't live on pure commission, so they work for someone who provides them with a base salary or a draw against future commissions.

Insurance companies pay the commissions, not the consumer. If consumers seek the agent's advice, they may pay a consulting fee.

With so little up-front financial promise, it is not surprising that the industry often employs recent college graduates who can live on a smaller income for a while. It is also not surprising that the industry has very high turnover.

Turnover is high because prospecting for new business can be daunting. So much negativity for relatively little money up front can really make a person miserable. Delivering the bad news of upsetting rate increases to disgruntled customers also takes thick skin.

Most brokers really do care about their clients. Many try very hard to lead their clients to less expensive plans. With our current population of often spoiled consumers, brokers get a lot of "push back" from their clients. Clients who refuse to change their ways, employee contribution or are closed to the idea of higher deductible plans, also contribute to the problem.

Brokers don't get paid until they close the sale. The client may be stalwart in their choice to pay a higher premium than needed. In this case, as often happens, the broker has put in many hours of work for which he may not receive compensation if the client leaves him. So, he gives in and writes you the plan you want instead of the plan he has recommended. When clients hire professionals for their advice and refuse to accept it, it puts the professional in an awkward position.

The flip side of the coin is the few brokers who routinely sell higher premium plans. The folks make their living by selling more expensive products that bring them higher commissions. This formula does not work in the consumer's favor when it comes to lower-priced health insurance plans. Logically, the lower the total cost of the premium, the lower the flat percent-based commission that the insurance agent receives.

Selling low-premium plans yields low commissions, so as an insurance agent there is less incentive to sell these plans. When a quality broker is offering to cut his own income to improve your company, it is wise for the client to heed this advice!

Let me give you an example of how much commission is riding on the employer's decision. For a twenty-person company in New Jersey that includes the dependents of those employees with families, I have seen total monthly costs for an HMO or PPO plan range from $15,000 to $40,000 in premiums! That means each year, that company is paying anywhere from $180,000 to $480,000 in premiums!

The insurance person that is making 5 percent on this plan receives $750 to $2,000 per month commission or $9,000 to $24,000 per year off of that account. There are significant incentives to sell high-end plans.

The example to which I am referring is an account that I personally prospected. I showed the employer all of the benefits of high-deductible health insurance and then ran the premiums. As a broker, I represent many companies, and I showed the customer the best coverage for the most frugal rates from all the providers in the state. With a high-deductible plan, the premiums dropped to between $6,000 and $16,000 per month with an annual cost of between $72,000 and $192,000 per year.

The savings of 60 percent over their current plan spoke volumes. If the employer put a $2,500 deductible on every person and a $5,000 deductible on each family, the total cost of the package yielded a savings of $108,000 to $288,000! Seems like a no-brainer choice to me!

The employer might even use a Health Reimbursement Account (HRA) to cover every employee's deductible. An HRA gives the employer the ability to accept the risk of all of the deductibles to protect his or her employees against suddenly high out-of-pocket costs.

This plan would cost the agent a significant amount of commission if he were to switch them down. The agent's commission would drop between $300 and $800 per month (a loss of commission of between $450 and $1,200 per month) or a total annual commission of between $3,600 and $9,600. That represents a decrease of 60 percent in income over the previous year.

Can you imagine what would happen if an insurance company's agents switched ten accounts to higher-deductible plans? That agent might fiscally cripple his employer! The agent would likely be fired.

In a commission-based business, you need to be an educated consumer to make sure you choose wisely.

 EHICs are willing to pay a licensed professional for his or her advice and direction to be sure that they receive money-saving advice that is in their best interests.

What logical reason could a business owner find not to offer a higher-deductible insurance policy for those employees who would benefit? The decisions that are made in buying health insurance are based on fear, and fear is illogical.

The only way to make logical decisions is to break apart the fear. When health insurance decisions are evaluated based on sound statistical data, the fear is significantly reduced.

In his book, *Deadly Spin*, Wendell Potter alludes to the profitability behind the insurance industry–sponsored fear mongering strategies. He outlines a series of fear mongering strategies employed by health insurance companies to keep the playing field highly profitable.

In the absence of logic, in the absence of an incentive system that compensates insurance sales professionals to uphold their fiduciary responsibility to the consumer, and in the absence of hard knowledge of retail prices, that prospect I mentioned never became a client. The company's CFO knew this was a good deal but played into the fears of her less-financially minded employees.

Chapter 9

Voluntary Benefits:
A Misnomer

Anytime you pay for something with your own money, it should be voluntary. The same goes for benefits. The added perk with employer-based benefits is that often the premiums are deducted on a pretax basis, which saves the employee and the employer taxes. In addition, the employer reliably pays the premiums, which keeps the policies in force longer.

Perhaps all benefits should be considered voluntary. You receive your benefits in lieu of salary, so you should choose how you wish to be compensated for the work that you do. One way or another, we pay for all of our benefits.

Voluntary benefits may include dental, vision, disability, and a variety of "dread disease" plans. They vary from employer to employer.

Voluntary benefits primarily protect the policyholder. They have taken a backseat to health insurance. Because health insurance premiums are so expensive, a lot of families have chosen to cancel policies where they themselves would be the financial beneficiaries in an effort to balance the family budget.

The following types of plans send cash to the policyholders' homes: disability (short term and long term), life insurance (whole or term), accident and hospitalization, and finally, "dread disease" insurance policies. Dread disease policies pay out in the event the policyholder is diagnosed with a serious illness, such as cancer. In each of the above-listed plans, the policyholder receives the monetary payout.

There is an enormous ongoing PR campaign to persuade healthy people to buy health insurance. There is very little coordinated effort by the various voluntary benefits industries to encourage people to protect their own cash flow.

When I have worked with clients who offer plans like disability or life insurance to their employees, I spend a lot of time reinforcing the need to continue to offer the plans. Some companies have very little interest because employees are skeptical of the benefits. People often tell me, "It sounds too good to be true." Or, "I haven't any money left after I pay for my health insurance." Employees are frequently so annoyed at paying such high premiums for health benefits they don't feel they use that they just say no to anything else.

Disability Insurance Protects You Against the Loss of Your Income

The insurance plans that benefit the individual are often difficult for the average consumer to understand. Most clients understand disability insurance (income insurance). They know that when their pay is turned off, disability insurance is what turns on their cash flow again.

Given the 3 percent risk of a hospitalization, many employees have no idea how expensive it is to get sick because they have never been really sick or hurt. It is often hard to explain that there are more costs associated with an illness or accident than simply medical costs. If you have never had a significant illness or injury, you may not realize that your medical insurance is not going to cover every expense associated with a medical disaster.

Clients are often confused about why any insurance would send them a check. And given how much they pay for health insurance, they are suspicious of the relatively low price tags of the various voluntary benefits.

One of the biggest hurdles that I face when helping clients choose benefits is the common belief that if you have medical insurance and anything goes medically wrong, all of your financial needs will be met by the health insurance provider.

EHICs take responsibility for protecting their family cash flow. They understand that health insurance is there to pay new medical bills and that most other types of insurance are the key to protecting your own financial solvency.

These days, a major illness or accident can cost a family that believes they have excellent medical insurance thousands of out-of-pocket dollars. The obvious additional expenses include deductibles and medical procedures that are only partially covered. Alternative therapy options are usually excluded from most traditional major medical plans.

There are many other expenses that happen when an accident or illness occurs. In the event of a diagnosis of cancer, for example, the whole family's balance shifts. You may have had two income earners, and now there is only one. However, that one earner is working part time. The primary earner is very likely going with the patient to doctor appointments, waiting through surgeries, and keeping the patient company in the hospital.

Did the patient have disability insurance?

Do you have life insurance?

After the caregiver has burned through vacation and sick time, he or she also may be eligible to go on FMLA, or the Family Medical Leave Act. He or she receives a reduced salary due to the Family Medical Leave Act, providing he or she has been with his or her current employer a minimum of twelve months. The FMLA payout is a reduced amount as compared with the caregiver's regular pay. If the family member or the caregiver supports his or her family on commissions, the income may just vanish.

If you have some short-term disability insurance, for a while, you may have some money coming into the home. If you are like most Americans, most every incoming dollar is accounted for as an outgoing expense. It does not take that long for a family to become insolvent when their predictable expenses are greater than their income. When finances head south, it is time to dip into savings, put big expenses on credit cards, or even worse, dip into retirement funds.

Other Sources of Income That Protect Your Assets When Illness or Accidents Happen

The plans that cover your family's needs are just as important, if not more important, than the health insurance plans. Hospitalization-only plans typically pay a daily benefit to the family between $100 and $300 and sometimes even $500. Benefits vary depending upon the coverage you purchased. The premiums are often less than $50–$100 per month for a couple.

Dread disease plans pay an incremental benefit if you have cancer, heart disease, or any of the dreadful diseases listed in the policy. They can pay between $100 and $300 for every day you are going through urgent care and $100 or so for the days that you are going through recuperative care. Dread disease policies also cost a couple about $50–$100 per month.

The benefits from these plans can financially save a family. The premiums are taken out of your salary pretax, and the benefits are usually paid to you tax free. Employers benefit because they don't pay FICA taxes on the pretax dollars. The family is relieved of some additional finance-related stress. The patient can focus on getting better. Voluntary benefits are designed to help you pay both the routine bills *and* the new and unexpected bills.

The unexpected bills come in all sorts of shapes and sizes. They might be little like parking, tolls, coffees, and food. You may find you have to rely on your car a lot more due to physical challenges during your recuperation, and be unable to use public transportation. Or the expenses can be significant. You may have to hire someone for a while to do the things around your home that you cannot do. You may need to hire caregivers for your children. You may need to move your family to a temporary residence closer to a faraway specialty treatment location. None of these expenses will be borne by your health insurance provider.

There is a common wisdom to keep three months' salary in the bank as a safety cushion in the event of some sort of disaster. In my career, I have met very few people who have actually achieved that goal. For many families, all these extra expenses may be enough to sink them financially.

Voluntary benefits are just as important as major medical benefits. Employers are doing the employees a disservice when voluntary benefits are not offered as part of a benefits plan.

For all benefits, education should be mandatory and participation should be voluntary. It's your money. You work hard to earn it. You should be allowed to decide how you spend it.

Chapter 10

Managing Predictable Costs

Budget: a mathematical confirmation of your suspicions.
—A. A. Latimer

Routine dental checkups and cleanings, prescriptions, and vision care are maintenance items that are predictable in nature. They are, or should be, planned expenses in your budget. Just like that oil change for your car, they are part of the cost of caring for your body.

If you take a monthly prescription, you know how you benefit from that therapy. You know that you will need certain prescriptions every month, just like you know that you should have a dental checkup twice a year.

These costs are predictable. There is no risk. In the absence of risk, there is no need for insurance.

An insurance policy is a "one-way contract." This means that in exchange for a specific premium, you are buying some sort of protection. The insurance company determines the terms of the contract, the benefit, and the premium. Most of us cannot negotiate any part of this contract. The information goes one way: from the insurance company to you. (In a two-way contract like a house sale, you could make a counteroffer.)

The insurance company is in this business to make money. The premiums are set based upon the likelihood that they will be paid. A young person is at very low risk of suddenly dying, so life insurance premiums are quite low. A person in his or her nineties is nearly at the end of his or her life span, and there is no price an insurance company will accept in exchange for a life insurance policy. This is because the likelihood they will have to pay out on the policy is very high.

In the case of dental, vision, and prescription insurance, prices are well established. Using actuarial tables, insurance companies know how much an average person at a certain age is going to need for average, noncatastrophic care. Let's look at these manageable costs one at a time.

Dental Plans

My health plan doesn't cover dental, so I enrolled my teeth as thirty-two dependents, each needing a complete physical once a year.
—Robert Brault

Insurance is designed to protect you against risk and there is not a lot of risk in dental care. It is expensive and most of us generally don't like to pay for expensive things that do not bring us great joy. You pay a lot of money and it may be very uncomfortable during the visit. But there is rarely a lot of financial risk. There may be a lot of cost, but most dentists can tell you up front what the cost will be.

The name alone—"plan" not "insurance"—should alert you to the fact that this is different. A dental plan is a discount plan that is designed to reduce and defray out-of-pocket costs. It rarely covers the entire list of services received.

The health insurance companies (and not you) know statistically what the costs are going to be for people in every demographic. They set the prices to be sure that they are profitable.

Dental plans are, for the most part, capped and managed. They are sometimes added to the maintenance component of your health insurance policy. You may have an exceptional year where your policy pays out more in a dental benefit than you pay in. Statistically, however, you will pay in more in premiums than your providers are likely to receive in benefits. To reduce their risk, your dental plan will likely have exclusions or limitations on how much will be paid for very costly procedures.

The primary advantage of plans where you go to a participating dentist is that rates they charge for their services have been negotiated lower on your behalf. From that perspective, you may save on your final cost to the dentist.

Again, the benefit is rarely more than the amount of collected premium because the plan knows the risk from actuarial tables.

Certain procedures may not be covered. This is because there is a risk that the cost will exceed the profitable parameters set by the health insurance companies in exchange for the premiums they are requesting.

A good example of a need that is frequently not covered is orthodontics. Braces can cost a few thousand to many thousands of dollars. The procedures are usually excluded as cosmetic. Cosmetic procedures are based on vanity, and insurance companies don't pay for vanity. They pay for disaster. Crooked teeth are not considered a disaster by an insurance company.

Large groups may have an orthodontic benefit built into a plan. The lifetime benefit is usually capped. That means that they will only pay out a finite amount. And, given coordinated benefits, even if you change employers or switch providers, they know how much already has been paid by your previous insurer.

Orthodontia is expensive but not risky. If you have ever had to cover the costs associated with orthodontia, you know that at the start of this long-term procedure you will have a visit with the orthodontist's financial manager.

The financial manager at the orthodontist's office reviews the predictable costs associated with their recommended solution to your problem. They will carefully explain to you all of the costs involved in getting the braces put on your teeth, and all of the services you can expect the orthodontist to include. You will then receive several payment options. You choose the plan that works best for you. You can also choose to decline their services.

When it comes to using a dental plan, either you go to a doctor who is willing to accept the contracted amount for certain procedures or you pay the whole price. With that said, it is becoming more and more common for the dentist to expect you to pay the balance between what your insurance pays and what they charge. They feel they charge a fair fee in exchange for services rendered.

You are paying the premiums, paying for all the noncovered procedures, and paying the balance due after the insurance paid a percent of the claim. The benefit will not exceed the premium, and more often than not, you are paying more because you are adding a layer of administrative costs. For most people, dental insurance is simply not worth the investment.

Not surprisingly, dentists can tell you the costs for any procedure very easily. Because health insurance companies are not universally expected to pay, there is complete transparency.

Costs are predictable and easy to understand. For that reason, it is very easy to do your homework and determine if the coverage you are considering will have any real value to you.

 EHICs don't like to waste money. It makes good sense to take care of your teeth and to try to head off expensive dental procedures. If you don't take good care of your teeth, only you suffer the consequences. It is not the role of the insurance company to pay for your negligence. EHICs have "skin in the game" and manage their oral health. This reduces the risk and expense associated with dental visits. Dental health premiums rarely offer EHICs value.

Prescription Plans

It is easy to get a thousand prescriptions but hard to get one single remedy.
—Chinese proverb

Prescription plans are rarely worth the investment. As with dental and health insurance, there is the same one-way contract and the same maintenance contract. Most people do not have access to how the fees for their insurance are determined.

Like dental plans, the maximum benefit in a prescription plan is usually capped and equal to no more than the total collected annual premium.

People who take monthly medications know that the therapy they need is vital to their well-being. Medications both treat and prevent illness. They also help you avoid developing more costly medical problems.[1]

Consider the following example. In New Jersey, one particular company offers two direct-to-consumer policies. The first has a prescription benefit; the second policy offers all the same benefits except there is no prescription coverage. Under the first policy, the prescription coverage is capped at $2,500, and the benefit is paid out at 50 percent of the cost of each prescription as it is redeemed. The difference in cost between the two plans is $2,495 per year for the plan with prescription coverage. In other words you will pay $5 less out-of-pocket for your medications if you fill $5000 worth of prescriptions with the prescription plan.

How can this be a good investment? If you don't need $5,000 worth of prescriptions each year, you are paying in premium with no chance of receiving the benefit in return.

Let's look at another example. Say you need to fill a prescription that costs $100. You might have a prescription plan that adds $200 to the basic plan each month. Your co-pay might be 50 percent for a brand-name drug. If the prescription costs $100, your benefit paid for the prescription was $50. Your co-pay is also $50. If that is the only prescription you fill this month, your total out-of-pocket expense for the prescription is $250!

The person without any prescription coverage, who paid cash for the prescription, paid $100. If that is the only prescription he or she buys this month, the total out-of-pocket cost is $100.

If you fill a $100 prescription every month for a year, it costs $1,200. If you fill that same prescription every month for a year with the prescription insurance, it really costs you $250 x 12, or $3,000. The work sheets at the back of the book can help you to determine if there is value for you with the prescription plan that you are being offered.

The question becomes, how much is your actual-out-of pocket monthly need? How much does your prescription cost? Not, how much is your co-pay, but rather, how much is the full retail price on the prescription? Given that prices can vary from store to store, how much is your retail price from four different stores?

EHICs do their homework before they fill a prescription. They have the phone numbers in their cell phones of four or five local pharmacies and call around to learn the cost *before* filling the prescription. If the prescription is going to be an ongoing expense, they also look online for pharmacies with lesser overhead that may charge less. EHICs always consider generic substitution as an option.

There is a common misconception that all drugs cost hundreds of dollars each month. In 2008, the average cost of a prescription was $71.69, with a generic costing on average $35.22 and a brand therapy costing $137.90.[2]

You can call around or look online and get different prices for the same product. One drugstore might have a preferential contract with a certain wholesaler who is promoting a certain product. So, for one month, a drug price at one pharmacy might be different from the cost at another pharmacy. The next month that could change. For the last few years, a national discount chain has had a promotion for three-dollar prescriptions. They claim that their bulk purchasing gives them extraordinary negotiating power with the wholesalers and the pharmaceutical companies.

In 2008, a *Consumer Reports* study of four specific prescription drugs found price variations of between $100 and $340, even when shopping within individual chain stores.[3] American consumers are not used to comparison shopping for drugs, so these price variations go largely unnoticed.

For the majority of people, these predictable costs are better managed by paying as you go. In the workbook section of this book, there is an easy guide to walk through about prescriptions. Some lucky people may know they benefit from having a prescription plan added to their policies, but most need to do some homework before knowing how it will play out.

Vision Plans

Very few employers offer vision plans any longer. In the world of manageable and predictable expenses, vision plans are not much better than discount plans. Retailers have found a way to capitalize on this market and know how to do so without compromising quality and safety.

This market is so competitively priced that the retailers offer optometry services and the ophthalmologists offer retail products. The prices are known and predictable. The corrective products come with all sorts of warranties and guarantees from both the retailers and the manufacturers. In fact, this is pretty much as close to a risk-free environment as you can get.

If you have a vision benefit, you will have to go to the provider and abide by the rules. Anything above the basic needs will be an additional cost.

Any serious eye injury or major illness is covered by your health insurance policy. Your eyes are indemnified against disaster in your health plan.

There is not a lot of risk associated with eyeglasses, so there is not a lot of reason to buy insurance.

Chapter 11

Managing Seemingly Unmanageable Costs

What if you really can't afford health insurance? If you cannot afford health insurance, then you likely do not currently pay for it. I am of the opinion that not everybody needs to have health insurance at all times.

What is the worst thing that might happen if you experience an accident or an illness and seek medical help during a time that you have no health insurance? The first thing that the doctor or hospital emergency room financial person will do is to ask you to pay for the services rendered. If you are like most Americans, you generally pay for your groceries at the store and for your oil change at the oil change place, so this will not come as much of a surprise.

If you have ample funds, there is an excellent probability that you will pull out the credit card or pay in cash and be done with it. If the costs are more than you have at hand, you may ask if you can pay some now and some later. If your accident or illness lands you in the hospital, things get a bit more complicated, but the theory remains the same: they expect you to pay.

So, the worst thing that happens is that you are expected to pay for services rendered. Already, I know that this thought is sending shivers up your spine. Why? *Because you have absolutely no idea what prices you will see on your bill.*

What Happens If You Can't Pay Your Medical Bills Immediately?

A few years ago, my brother-in-law fell off a horse he was riding and broke both his arm and his leg. It took a herculean effort to make him go to the doctor because he did not have health insurance at the time. After suffering significantly for two days, he did seek medical attention and ended up with a two-night hospital admission to have his broken arm and broken leg set surgically.

Then came the scary part: the bill. After some negotiation, they reduced the inflated numbers usually submitted to the providers who pay only a fraction of what they are billed. The price tag dropped by half. They set up financing, and for five years—like a car payment—he paid off the amount.

High-deductible health insurance would have been a good choice for him. But he had chosen not to buy health insurance because, to him, it looked as if his only choice was to pay $400 a month to have an HMO or PPO. What if he had been offered a hundred-dollar-per-month plan that had a high deductible? He could likely have afforded it and would likely have bought that plan.

Most people who can't afford health insurance are very good people with families, and the $700–$1,500 (or more) per-month price tag is daunting. High-deductible plans are not always presented in the most palatable manner. People fear they won't be able to pay the deductible all at once.

This type of plan may not be the right one for everyone but for the young and healthy, it is much better to have something than to have nothing.

But let's say you elect to have no coverage at all and fall off a horse. The laws protect you as long as you make good-faith efforts to pay the money you owe every month. You may only pay twenty dollars or you may pay a hundred dollars per month or more. Whatever you negotiate with the medical facility to pay, as long as you do pay every month, your credit will be fine and your providers will work with you.

If you don't have health insurance and you can't pay your medical bills, you can go bankrupt. No one wants that, but if things are so bad that you can't afford a high-deductible plan and you can't pay your medical obligations, you are also likely struggling on other financial fronts. You may have too much debt on your credit cards and you may already be feeling the pressure of financial obligations you cannot meet. No one likes bankruptcy, but if you have no choice, there are laws to protect you.

Let me make it clear: I don't agree with not having health insurance: Having no health insurance at all is very risky.

How You Are Conditioned by the Health Insurance Industry

We have been conditioned by the health insurance providers to buy health insurance or perish. Only when you understand that you have been nursed, raised, and fed on their corporate spin can you can rein in your out-of-control, out-of-pocket medical costs.

It is not your fault. When people are downsized or lose their jobs, the first thing that they fear is losing their health insurance. It seems to me that this should be fourth or fifth on the list of worries.

If you lose your job, shouldn't your first worry be, do you have the money to pay the mortgage or rent? After that comes, how can you keep the family fed and the lights on? Do you have enough funds to float your family's basic needs until you find the next job? Your biggest concern *should not be*, in the event your child gets a cold or the flu, will your doctors get paid immediately?

Amazingly, the conditioning is so complete that our personal needs take a backseat to our perceived higher priority need to have health insurance.

You Are Manipulated into Buying More Health Insurance Than You Need

There is no PR campaign, day in and day out, telling you, scaring you, or selling you about keeping your family fed or housed. There is no organized machine designed to keep you aware that missed mortgage or rent payments may have disastrous consequences. There is no multimillion-dollar for-profit-funded organization constantly flooding the airwaves with messages to "save your money" and "spend prudently" to make your funds last between jobs.

When you become an educated consumer of health insurance, you will make a budget. That budget should include all your basic costs, such as your housing, utilities, and communication expenses. It should also include insurance premiums and savings. If you create a financial buffer for yourself, you can protect your family.

By self-insuring your deductible, you learn that there is a tremendous financial upside to budgeting for your more predictable, manageable expenses.

Buying health insurance is like hiring the health insurance provider to manage your day-to-day medical expenses on your behalf. It is simply too expensive for the average small employer, its employees, or the individual consumer to pay for services they don't really need.

Chapter 12

Conclusion:
The Power of the Educated Consumer

Clearly, the health insurance industry likes the status quo, so it discourages change. The federal government is seemingly powerless to make any significant changes to address the growing health care concerns. That leaves the individual consumers, the human resources professionals, and the CEOs, CFOs, and COOs of corporations with the power to bring on change.

At the start of this book, I listed some changes that would help alleviate the consumer's pain:

1. Full health insurance plans in paper mailed to every consumer, outlining coverage and exclusions in a simple language that a layman can understand;
2. Universal common claim forms to reduce administrative waste;
3. Published contracted prices;
4. Annually published actuarial and risk tables;
5. Transparency through standardization and a universal template of policy coverage and explanations;
6. Optional participation in group health plans; and
7. Mandatory at-work access to policy educators who will answer questions and explain coverage.

As consumers, the large corporations and human resource professionals have the power to make some of these changes happen. They can demand paper policies be sent to all of their employees. They can also create a template of easy-to-understand language and require that providers put their policies into a standard format. Finally, they can mandate education and access to policy educators to answer questions and explain coverage. If the first company will not work with you, the educated consumer has the power to choose a new provider that will work with you.

When the corporations bring on these changes, the news media can choose to write the stories that reinforce these successes. The stories can be the catalyst for smaller companies to flex their muscles. This is how grassroots movements gain popularity. The providers who want your business will work with you and the inflexible providers will lose your business.

Change happens slowly. Our personal situation is the same as our neighbors' in some ways and different in others.

By becoming an EHIC, you are becoming an agent for change. Not only will you keep more money in your pocket but you will become part of a movement for change. If enough people embrace this approach to their insurance, the companies will see their bottom line shift.

Let's see what the policy makers come up with at that point. For now, if we don't embrace taking control of our health insurance … you can expect more of the same.

Chapter 13

The Workbook

Absent information, the (free) market cannot work. How can people choose effectively if they lack the information needed to make intelligent choices?[1]

The following is what I believe to be the correct plan for consumers based on their personal conditions. Of course, you need to look at your own personal circumstances before making a choice.

PPO and POS—No one! (That was easy.) It is the best moneymaker for the insurance company, and you are stuck with higher co-pays and higher out-of-pocket maximums.

HMO—There are several types of people who should consider HMOs.

- People with ongoing chronic conditions requiring more than one doctor visit per quarter.
- Young families planning on having children or who have at least two young children under age six.
- Individuals who have been warned by their health care providers that they should be watched carefully for fear of a certain health condition.

High-Deductible Health Insurance—Qualified Plans Only

- Younger and otherwise healthy individuals and couples who usually only seek medical attention for regular checkups.

- Families and couples with significant income who can benefit from $3,050/$6,150 pretax-savings tax deductions.
- Individuals and couples looking to retire in the next ten to fifteen years with no underlying illness. (They can use the tax-free savings to further reinforce their financial security at retirement.)
- Individuals, couples, and families who have chosen to be uninsured in light of economic and family budgeting realities. (Better to have some protection than none at all in the event of medical disaster.)

As an educated consumer, you can save money in two ways. First, just pay for the few random visits to the doctors you want who fall outside your network. Second, with qualified high-deductible health care plans, annual preventative care is paid at the HMO co-pay rate before the deductible is satisfied.

Consumer-Driven Health Care: Why Do I Want to Pay for High-Deductible Health Insurance?

Let's be sure we are all on the same page as to how consumer-driven health care plans or high-deductible health insurance plans are supposed to work. High-deductible health plans are the indemnity plans of yesteryear.

High-deductible plans come in two forms—qualified and nonqualified. A qualified plan conforms to federal regulations and offers a finite amount of risk to the consumer. An unqualified plan offers risks to the consumer that may be significantly greater than the value to the consumer. If the plan has a $15,000 out-of-pocket risk, that plan is not "qualified"—it is a poor choice, and I would advise against anyone buying it. The low premiums are too much of a trade-off for the out-of-pocket risk associated with a major accident or illness.

Let us say that you have a qualified high-deductible health plan. A qualified plan in 2011 has a minimum deductible of $1,200 for an individual and a minimum deductible of $2,400 for a couple. (If you are an individual with a $1,000 deductible, you do not have a qualified plan.) It also has a maximum out-of-pocket risk of $5,950 for an individual. The maximum out-of-pocket risk is $11,900 for a family. If you have a maximum out-of-pocket risk greater than that amount, you do not have a qualified plan.[2]

With a qualified plan, you may open a high-deductible savings account. Each year, an individual may contribute $3,050, and a family may contribute $6,150.[3] These contributions are in pretax dollars, so right away, they are worth more than the actual figures you see. These tax-free dollars may be used to pay for "qualified expenses." (For a complete list of qualified expenses, each year the government publishes *Publication 502*.[4])

Please note that I am not talking about a health care reimbursement account here, which often has a yearly "use-it-or-lose-it" clause. Money saved in a high-deductible health care account can be carried over from year to year. This means that at the end of the year, all the money you have saved (redirected perhaps from monies not spent on premiums with high administrative fees) can be put toward next year or taken as taxable income.

 EHICs think about the risk-benefit ratio and the tax laws when considering health insurance. Unless they have no assets and nothing to lose, having no insurance is a very risky proposition. EHICs consult their accountants or tax professionals to be sure they maximize on all health insurance and tax benefits and deductions.

Answering the Naysayers

When logical options are presented, it is sometimes hard to see through the misconceptions that are firmly planted in our minds. Fear takes a very strong hold on many people's ability to understand risk.

"Oh no, that's not how it would work at all!" I can hear the naysayers now. There are many common excuses offered by the general population as to why this would not work:

1. "My employer pays most of my premium, so that isn't a real example!"

   (Answer: You are getting this benefit in lieu of actual income. Even though you might not see what is being paid, the cost is real. You would care if your check was increased by the actual costs paid. Your employer cares because that cost prevents him or her from being able to pay you more.)

2. "If I had an extra $3,000, there is no way I am going to let it sit in a savings account. I have bills to pay!"

   (Answer: The choice to save is yours. The best way to achieve this savings is to make the deposit directly into a qualified pretax savings account at the time your paycheck is issued. If you draw the funds, you will have to pay taxes at that time. If you leave them there, you have earned a return equal to your tax rate. And, if there is an accident or major illness, there is more money to spend on qualified expenses. Part of managing your budget is being responsible for your spending.)

3. "I cannot control myself and save like that."

   (Answer: Then do not complain about your high premiums. If you abdicate responsibility for your own spending, you have no right to complain about those who take your money.)

4. "You are making up numbers to make this look real— but I know medical costs are skyrocketing, and I will go broke if I have to pay for my medical costs as I go!"

   (Answer: Please feel free to look up any of the references cited. Costs may be increasing but the research here shows that the health insurance companies are adding significantly to those costs. These increased costs go largely undetected because there is no coordinated effort of a diverse group of health care practitioners and service providers to educate the public and create a counter spin campaign to negate the health insurance company's spin.)

5. And look out, here come the insurance companies. "You offer these plans," they will say, "but no one wants them."

(Answer: The truth is that these types of plans are not nearly as profitable for the insurance companies as PPOs and POSs. So, they spin out a message that people don't want the products they offer because they are the least profitable. They push the consumer toward the products they offer that make the health insurance companies the most profit.)

It is really easy to fall into the trap of thinking everyone needs the "maintenance contract" as much as we need the "indemnity contract." We have all grown up with the maintenance contract. This change may feel as uncomfortable as driving on the left-hand side of the road.

Examples to Frame Your Thinking for the Work Sheets

As an example, imagine a company that manufactures clothing and has twenty employees. The policies might break out as follows:

	Maintenance Plan HMO PPO/POS	High-Deductible Plan $2,500 deductible
Single $250 $400		$150
1-parent family $400 $650		$325
Husband/wife $450 $850		$275
2-parent family $650 $1100		$550

Assuming the company has five employees who fall neatly into each stage-of-life family category, the total monthly premiums would be as follows:

5	Single employees
5	1-parent family
5	Husband/wife employees
<u>5</u>	2-parent family employees
20	Total number of policies that will be written

If all twenty employees bought the same type of plan, the premiums each month break out as follows:

20 employee HMO	$7,850 per month
PPO/POS plan	$15,000 per month
High deductible	$6,250 per month

The employer benefits from a savings of $1,600 per month for the company that moves to high-deductible health care from an HMO plan, or $19,200 per year.

The savings are even greater if the company moves from the higher cost plans (PPO/POS $15,000–$6,250 for the high-deductible plan) of $8,480 per month, or $101,760 per year.

Example # 1: High-Deductible Health Insurance, Single

The employee pays 30 percent of his health care premium for his high-deductible plan which costs $150 per month, or $1,800 per year. His 30 percent contribution is $45 per month, or $540 per year.

His guaranteed monthly premium expense is $45. With only a 3 percent risk of hospitalization, it is unlikely he will spend the whole deductible. It is most likely he may pay for one or two visits to an MD ($75 per visit x 2 visits = $150) and maybe get a generic prescription for $10. So, his real annual cost is likely to be about $540 health insurance and $160 medical costs, or a total of $700!

Example #2: HMO Policy

That same employee has a $250 per month HMO, for which he contributes 30 percent or $75 per month. He has the same two visits for which he pays a $50 co-pay and $15 for a prescription. His total annual cost is $75 x 12 months for his health insurance premium = $900 + $115 for two doctor visits and a prescription: $1015!

Example # 3: POS/PPO

That same employee pays 30 percent of the now $400 monthly premium, or $120 per month. He pays $60 to see the doctor of his choice and, on two occasions, $15 for the same tier one prescription. His total annual cost is $120 x 12 for medical = $1,440 + ($60 x 2) for medical visits and $15 for prescription: $1,575!

The savings are obvious: when the employee looks at the numbers, a $2,500 high-deductible plan will cost $700 per year, the HMO will cost about $1,015 per year, and the PPO/POS will cost $1,575 per year! Given a 3 percent risk of hospitalization, that employee can be insured for about half of what he is likely paying now. The savings are even more dramatic for single-parent families, husband-and-wife households, and families.

In the far less likely event of a hospitalization, that employee may well be looking at paying $2,500. But it does not all have to be paid that day. As long as good faith efforts to pay are made, that employee might pay off the deductible at $25 or $50 or $100 per month over the next few years. As the Educated Health Insurance Consumer knows, there is a 97 percent chance this will not happen to you this year. So, don't pay for something you don't need, and don't buy *that* insurance until you have worked out the numbers.

 EHICs understand that they do not need to pay annually the full face value of risk into a system that is designed to increase shareholder value. They take responsibility budget and pay for routine, predictable, and manageable health care costs.

Your Needs and Your Background Research

As an informed consumer, you need to gather some key information at hand before the decision-making process begins. There are several key pieces of data you will need to collect from your own personal data archives.

Use the following pages to understand your current costs and needs. You may choose to photocopy the pages if you have multiple plan options. If both you and your spouse are employed and offered benefits through both employers, you will want to compare both sets of plans. Some employers may offer to "buy you out" of your health insurance if you will go onto your spouse's insurance, so you may want to ask them about that. It could mean some extra money in your family budget.

This section is a look backward at your personal and family history of medical expenses. It is the baseline against which all other information will be compared. There may not be enough room for all answers in this workbook; duplicate pages as needed.

1.   How much money did you spend on each member of the family last year for medical service provider co-pays?

Adult #1:_____

Adult #2:_____

Child #1:_____

Child #2:_____

Child #3:_____

2.   How much money did you spend last year on prescription copays? What is the "cash" price?

Adult #1:_____/_____

Adult #2:_____/_____

Child #1:_____/_____

Child #2:_____/ _____

Child #3:_____/_____

3.   If anyone is on routine medicines, list them here:
Patient name   Drug name   Frequency   taken   (times   per
day)

_____

_____

_____

_____

_____

_____

4.   How much was your current total personal contribution
to your health insurance premium? (If spouse is on a different
plan, be sure to review both plans and list separately.)

Plan 1: Cost per pay: $_____ per month: $_____per year: $_____

Plan 2: Cost per pay: $_____ per month: $_____per year: $_____

5.   Call each of your family's *personally* preferred health
care providers, your GP, your pediatrician, allergists,
ophthalmologists, specialists seen routinely, OB, and so on. Ask
them how much they charge a cash-paying patient for an office
visit.

| | *Cash* cost per visit | Number of your visits last year |
Provider name:		
_____	$_____	#_____
_____	$_____	#_____
_____	$_____	#_____
_____	$_____	#_____
_____	$_____	#_____
_____	$_____	#_____

6.   How much was your employer's contribution to your health care costs? (This information will become mandatory for you to view in 2014 and will be on your pay stub. It is good to know now.)

Plan 1: Cost per pay: $_____ per month: $____per year: $____

Plan 2: Cost per pay: $_____ per month: $____per year: $____

Room for additional notes and questions:

Questions to Ask of Your Employer(s):

1.   How much was last year's total cost for your family's coverage?_____

2.   How much is this year's policy going to cost you, and how much are you paying into the plan?_____
_____

3.   Please review the specific changes of this plan as compared to the plan that is currently ending.
_____
_____
_____

4.   How much is the deductible, and what services are not applied to the deductible?_____
_____
_____
_____

5.   If you go to a doctor who is not part of your plan or who accepts only cash, how do you submit a courtesy copy of the   receipt   for   credit   toward   your deductible?_____
_____
_____
_____

6.   How does this health insurance policy define a preexisting condition? (It may be totally different from what you expect.) _____
_____
_____

Health Insurance Plan Options

Benefit	Plan 1: HMO	Plan 2: PPO/POS	Plan 3: HDHI
In-network OOP* maximum	$_____	$_____	$_____
Out-of-network OOP maximum	$_____	$_____	$_____
Do co-pays apply to OOP maximums?	Y/N	Y/N	Y/N
Deductible / person	$_____	$_____	$_____
Deductible /year	$_____	$_____	$_____
Is plan "qualified"?	Y/N		

PRIMARY CARE

	Plan 1: HMO	Plan 2: PPO/POS	Plan 3: HDHI
Primary care co-pay	$_____	$_____	$_____

Preferred Providers:

	Plan 1: HMO	Plan 2: PPO/POS	Plan 3: HDHI
Does deductible have to be met before co-pay?	Y/N	Y/N	Y/N
Do reasonable and customary (R&C) charges apply?	Y/N	Y/N	Y/N

If yes, call customer service and request a copy of the charges.

Nonpreferred Providers:

	Plan 1: HMO	Plan 2: PPO/POS	Plan 3: HDHI
Does deductible have to be met before co-pay?	Y/N	Y/N	Y/N
Do reasonable and customary (R&C) charges apply?	Y/N	Y/N	Y/N

If yes, call customer service and request a copy of the charges.

List your family doctors who are preferred providers for each plan:

_____ _____ _____
_____ _____ _____
_____ _____ _____
_____ _____ _____
_____ _____ _____
_____ _____ _____
_____ _____ _____

110

SPECIALISTS:

Specialist co-pay $_____ $_____ $_____

Preferred Providers:
Does deductible have to
be met before co-pay?   Y/N   Y/N   Y/N
Do reasonable and customary
(R&C) charges apply?   Y/N   Y/N   Y/N
 If yes, call customer service and request a copy of the charges.
Nonpreferred Providers:
Does deductible have to
be met before co-pay?   Y/N   Y/N   Y/N
Do reasonable and customary
(R&C) charges apply?   Y/N   Y/N   Y/N
 If yes, call customer service and request a copy of the charges.

List your family doctors who are preferred providers for each plan:

_____ _____ _____
_____ _____ _____
_____ _____ _____
_____ _____ _____
_____ _____ _____
_____ _____ _____
_____ _____ _____

Routine physicals covered? Y/N   Y/N   Y/N
        Cost? $_____ $_____ $_____
Routine eye exams covered? Y/N   Y/N   Y/N
        Cost? $_____ $_____ $_____

Labs and x-rays $_____ $_____ $_____
Emergency room visit $_____ $_____ $_____
Chiropractic $_____ $_____ $_____
Ambulance $_____ $_____ $_____
Maternity $_____ $_____ $_____
Psychiatric $_____ $_____ $_____

Surgery pre-cert   Y/N   Y/N   Y/N

Dental Plan Options

Benefit	Plan 1	Plan 2
Annual coverage maximum / person	$_____	$_____
Annual deductible / person	$_____	$_____
Annual deductible / family	$_____	$_____
Orthodontic coverage?	Y/N	Y/N
If yes, lifetime maximum	$_____	$_____
TMJ coverage?	Y/N	Y/N
If yes, lifetime maximum	$_____	$_____

Indicate Coverage:

Endodontics	Y/N	Y/N
Periodontics	Y/N	Y/N
Oral surgery	Y/N	Y/N
Major restorative services	Y/N	Y/N
Prosthodontics	Y/N	Y/N

		List per person the total dental
New benefits		spent in past three years:
Cost per pay period	$_____	20__ $_____
Cost per month	$_____	20__ $_____
Cost per year	$_____	20__ $_____

Expected major work for family
due for the next year:

Call dentist and ask how
much each procedure will cost:

1._____$_____
2._____$_____
3._____$_____

Call insurance company and ask how much for each procedure will be
covered for each of the above known needs:

	Plan 1	Plan 2
1._____	$_____	$_____
2._____	$_____	$_____
3._____	$_____	$_____

Is the dental benefit worth the expense to you? Y/N

Prescription Cost Comparison

Take the information from the "Needs and Background Research" page and complete the following work sheet for each member of the family taking any prescription therapy. Call around to a variety of pharmacies to find out the *cash* price. (Don't forget to ask if they have any member discounts. You may get a better price if you join some sort of a membership club.)

List your local pharmacies and their phone numbers:

1._____ (____)_____
2._____ (____)_____
3._____ (____)_____
4._____ (____)_____

Patient name:_____
Drug:_____
Monthly cost $_____ $_____ $_____

Pharmacy #1_____ #2_____ #3_____

Patient name:_____
Drug:_____
Monthly cost $_____ $_____ $_____

Pharmacy #1_____ #2_____ #3_____

Patient name:_____
Drug: _____
Monthly cost $_____ $_____ $_____

Pharmacy #1_____ #2_____ #3_____

Patient name: _____

Drug: _____

Monthly cost $_____ $_____ $_____

 Pharmacy #1_____ #2_____ #3_____

Patient name:

Drug:

Monthly cost $_____ $_____ $_____

 Pharmacy #1_____ #2_____ #3_____

Total Predictable Costs for Monthly Prescriptions:
 Patient   Drug   Monthly Cash Price
1._____ _____ $_____
2._____ _____ $_____
3._____ _____ $_____
4._____ _____ $_____
5._____ _____ $_____

Cost of prescription plan for previous year $____

Cost of your co-pays for prescriptions for previous year $____

Premium for new prescription plan / month $____

                                        Per year $____

Co-pays for predictable prescriptions/ month $____

                                        Per year $____

Is there value in paying for the prescription plan this year?

_____

_____

Voluntary Benefit Costs and Options

Major medical insurance is designed to take the sting out of all the medical bills you may incur in the event that you or a family member is diagnosed with a disastrous illness or has a terrible accident.

Voluntary benefits look at the "your private bills and can't you pay them" risk. Too often, I talk with people who do not realize that when they get sick or hurt, not only will there be some additional medical bills arriving in the door, but the old, familiar bills that compromise the family budget continue to show up.

The average person often puts unexpected expenses on credit cards or uses the rent or mortgage money to pay the new bills. This can leave nothing to pay the rent or mortgage. Voluntary benefits are designed to help fill the financial gap that can occur at this point. Here are some things you need to consider:

1. What is the necessary income to cover your routine financial outflow each month? (Add up car payments and expenses, mortgage/rent, utilities, communication, food, child care, etc.)
    $ _____
2. How many months of savings do you have to meet that commitment? (In other words, if you need $4,000, do you have it in an accessible bank account? Do you have $8,000 for two months of cash flow?)_____
3. For how many months can you keep your bills paid if you are not working full time due to an illness or an accident by yourself or your spouse or child?

    _____

If you do not have three months of liquid savings on hand, it is best to consider some sort of personal income financial protection, aka disability.

1. Does your employer offer a disability plan?_____
2. Do you participate in it?_____
3. How much money do you get each month from that plan if you are disabled?_____

4.   How long does the plan go for (six months, one year, two years, or indefinitely)? _____

5.   How does that plan define disability?

_____

_____

6.   Does your state or union provide disability?_____

7.   If yes, how much and for how long?_____

8.   How does that plan define disability?

_____

_____

9.   Does your employer offer you access to disability that you can pay for yourself?_____

10.   If yes, do you buy this protection for yourself and for your family?_____ How much do you pay each year and for how long a benefit period?_____

11.   How does that plan define disability?

_____

_____

12.   Do you have any disability protection personally and/or privately?_____

13.   If yes, how much and for how long?_____

14.   How does that plan define disability?

_____

_____

As long as you have after-tax income through disability equal to two-thirds of your income for a year, you will most likely survive most unexpected accidents and illnesses with your personal financial assets intact. If you do not have that protection, you may be taking a bigger gamble than you realize.

Dread Disease Policies

As I mentioned, after a significant illness or hospitalization, your regular expenses come in, and so do extra new and unexpected expenses. So, you will likely need more cash flow than just disability. There are many providers and types of benefits that can augment your cash flow without compromising disability income laws. These policies pay cash to your family based on the severity of the accident or illness. You can use this cash to augment your income at a time when your expenses may increase. This is insurance where you are the beneficiary, not the doctor or the hospital, and it complements your disability policy or policies.

Voluntary benefits include but are not limited to accident protection, hospital protection, cancer or heart disease protections, and so on. To be clear, if you are diagnosed with cancer and you have a policy that sends you cash when you have a diagnosis of cancer, it is called a "cancer policy." If you have hospital protection and a covered member of your family is admitted to hospital, it is called a "hospital policy."

There are other diagnoses that can cause expenses to increase, such as stroke, heart disease, or cancer.

The types of plans vary, but in my experience, the risk of unexpected expenses increases when you hit the hospital. So, I encourage my clients to have some sort of cash flow protection that is activated by a hospital admission. The rates vary, so you need to do your homework. These are taken into consideration below:

1. How much does the policy pay to your family upon hospital admission?_____
2. How much does the policy pay to your family for each additional night in the hospital?_____
3. How long does the policy continue to pay?_____
4. What are the preexisting conditions clauses?

     _____

     _____

5. Does the policy cover you for rehabilitative care?____
6. If yes, how much and for how long?_____
7. How do you file a claim?

     _____

8. What is (are) the policy number(s) and providers?

     _____

     _____

9. Is there a death benefit?_____
10. If yes, how much? Are your beneficiaries up to date?_____
11. Did you list these plans in your will?
12. Who is your agent, and what is his or her contact information?

_____

_____

13. Is the policy guaranteed renewable?_____
14. Is the policy portable?_____
15. When and how might the premiums change?

_____

16. What are the other benefits of the policy (or policies)?

<u>Medical Treatment</u>   <u>Payout/Event_____</u>

- _____
- _____
- _____
- _____
- _____
- _____

If you have disability protection equal to two-thirds of your income and voluntary benefits that pay \$100–\$300 per day during active illness or major accident, you are likely in a better position to protect your personal financial assets.

Predictable Cost Management Summary

Predictable costs are just that—predictable. You may not like them, but you can budget for them. You may not want to budget for them, but there is no risk associated with them that requires insurance. So, there is no point in trying to buy insurance to cover them.

Person   <u>Annual cost</u> <u>Monthly cost</u>

Dental Care:

1._____   \$_____   \$_____
2._____   \$_____   \$_____
3._____   \$_____   \$_____
4._____   \$_____   \$_____

Prescriptions:

1._____ $_____ $_____
2._____ $_____ $_____
3._____ $_____ $_____
4._____ $_____ $_____

Disability:

1._____ $_____ $_____
2._____ $_____ $_____
3._____ $_____ $_____
4._____ $_____ $_____

Voluntary Benefits:
Life insurance:

1._____ $_____ $_____
2._____ $_____ $_____
3._____ $_____ $_____
4._____ $_____ $_____

Hospital protection: $_____ $_____
Cancer protection: $_____ $_____
Heart protection: $_____ $_____

Others:

_____ $_____ $_____
_____ $_____ $_____
_____ $_____ $_____

Health Insurance
Premium contribution: $_____ $_____
Co-pays

1._____ $_____ $_____
2._____ $_____ $_____
3._____ $_____ $_____
4._____ $_____ $_____

Total predictable and manageable costs:

$_____/month $_____/year

Those numbers may very well intimidate you. The cost of protecting ourselves from disaster while managing our health can be very overwhelming. The figures may represent a bigger portion of your budget than you realized. Not knowing these answers does not reduce the risks. Not planning, however, may result in the loss of everything.

Suggested Reading

The following are excellent books that discuss health care issues in depth. Each author offers an amazing amount of excellent research and information to the reader. These books will further enable you to understand the current health care landscape.

Who Killed Health Care?: America's $2 Trillion Medical Problem— and the Consumer-Driven Cure, Regina Herzlinger. (New York: McGraw-Hill, 2007)

Deadly Spin: An Insurance Company Insider Speaks Out on How Corporate PR Is Killing Health Care and Deceiving Americans, Wendell Potter. (New York: Bloomsbury Press, 2010)

The Innovator's Prescription: A Disruptive Solution for Health Care, Clayton M. Christensen. (New York: McGraw-Hill, 2009)

Glossary[1]

Affiliation Period. The amount of time a new plan member must wait before being eligible for health care coverage, imposed by the health plan and not an employer. This waiting period is not usually longer than three months. It is at the employers discretion.

Actuarial Tables. A table of statistical data that is used to determine risk and prices for insurance products, relative to risk or payout. Usually, the lower the risk that the company will pay out on the policy, the lower the premium. The greater the risk that the insurance company will be expected to pay out on the policy, the higher the insurance premium. Actuarial tables are created and read by professionals known as actuaries.

Agent. An agent is a person or business that is authorized to act on another's behalf. In insurance, a person who represents a single specific company at a specific time is acting as an agent for that insurance company. An insurance professional is "appointed" to an agency by way of a contractual agreement.

Beneficiary. The person or group that receives benefits, profits, or advantages of an insurance policy. The person designated as the recipient of funds. In health insurance, while the consumers may benefit from the medical products and services received, they are not the beneficiaries of the payments and are thus not the beneficiaries of their health insurance policy.

Broker. A person who functions as an intermediary between two or more parties in negotiating agreements, bargains, or contracts is brokering the policy. In health insurance, a person who represents many insurance companies at the same time is a health insurance broker. Once a plan is chosen, the broker then acts as an agent representing the carrier.

Balance Billing. When doctors and hospitals charge patients the difference between their fees and the amounts the insurance company paid.

Capitated Payment. A set payment to a health care provider for a certain amount of time or type of treatment regardless of how much care the individual gets or needs. The provider's financial incentive is to deliver as few services as possible. The opposite of capitated payments are fee-for-service payments. Often the provider does not know the exact amount of the expected compensation or the capitated payment that any given plan will pay for any service within any negotiated contract until the payment is received.

Carrier. The insurance company offering a health insurance policy is referred to as your insurance carrier or "carrier" for short.

Catastrophic Coverage. Insurance designed to protect an individual from having to pay very high out-of-pocket costs. Catastrophic coverage usually begins after the person has spent a predetermined amount called a deductible. Often referred to as "high-deductible" policies, catastrophic health coverage is a true insurance policy that is designed to protect you against financial disaster and generally costs up to half the annual cost of managed care policies.

Catastrophic Limit. Also referred to as an out of pocket maximum, the most amount of money an individual will have to pay out of pocket during a given period of time for medical services. After the person has reached the catastrophic limit, a higher level of coverage begins, though he or she may still have to pay some portion of health care costs. Not all out-of-pocket costs may count toward the catastrophic limit, the plan should cover the rest of your medical costs. You may call customer service to learn your limits for all out-of-pocket expenses related to your particular plan.

Certificate of Insurance. The printed description of the benefits and coverage provisions forming the contract between a person and his or her carrier, which details what the plan covers, what it does not, and dollar limits. The card that is wallet size and carried with consumers is evidence of a certificate of coverage.

Certificate of Credible Coverage. This is a letter that a customer receives at the end of a contract with a health insurance provider that certifies previous health insurance coverage for a specific amount of time during which the policy was in force. It may be requested by a new plan provider to prove uninterrupted coverage and to prevent denial of coverage or rolling effective dates for preexisting conditions. These letters should be kept in a safe location, as they are frequently required when switching providers. If a letter does not come to a customer, the customer may call customer service to receive a copy of their letter.

Claim. An itemized bill submitted to an insurance company invoicing the carrier for services or benefits a plan member received.

COBRA. The Consolidated Omnibus Budget Reconciliation Act (COBRA) is a federal law that guarantees employees and their families who lose their employer-sponsored health coverage—due to termination of employment, death, divorce, or other circumstances—the right to purchase continued coverage under the employer's group health plan for specific periods of time. Qualified individuals are required to pay the entire premium for coverage plus an administrative fee, up to 102 percent of the cost of the plan.

Coinsurance. The portion of the cost of care you are required to pay after your health plan pays. Usually, it is a percentage of the amount approved by the insurer, and it should have a "cap," or maximum out-of-pocket expense risk, for the contract year.

Conversion Policy. An employer-sponsored group health policy can be converted to an individual policy with the same insurance company, much like COBRA.

Covered Expenses. Major medical insurance policies cover doctor's office visits, lab expenses, hospital charges, and similar ordinary and necessary medical expenses.

Community Rating. A way to set insurance premiums that is based on the claims experience of people in a like group of applicants. With community rating, each policyholder's premium is based on the average cost of the entire pool—healthy and sick mixed together—and is not determined by each individual's age or health status. The opposite of community rating is "risk-based" rating.

Comprehensive. Insurance coverage that covers all conceivable health costs. Universal health insurance plans, including the state-sponsored plans, may not be comprehensive coverage.

Contracted Pricing. Once you have purchased a health insurance plan, your fees and costs will be paid out at the rate negotiated with each contracted provider. The specific payment is often blinded to both the provider of the product and services, as well as to the customer. Usual and customary prices are shown, but they do not often represent the actual contracted payment.

Co-payment. A set amount you are required to pay for each medical service you receive, such as a visit to your doctor, use of lab services, a hospital visit, or a prescription.

Cost Sharing. Co-pays and out-of-pocket costs for medical care or the portion of medical care that you pay yourself, such as a coinsurance or deductible, are how consumers are asked to bear the burden and share the cost of ever-increasing medical care. Sharing in the cost of premiums is called "cost shifting."

Cost Tiers. A system that insurance plans use to set drug coverage cost sharing. Generic drugs are generally on the first, least expensive tier of the plan's formulary, followed by brand-name drugs and then specialty drugs, with each subsequent tier requiring higher cost sharing.

Deductible. The amount of health care expenses you must pay – at the reduced, agreed, negotiated rate -before your health insurer begins to pay. Deductibles may be affiliated with a calendar year or a plan year if your health insurance plan year does not align with the calendar year. There may be a separate deductible for prescription products that is in addition to the deductible for health products and services.

Denial of Coverage. A refusal by your insurer to pay for medical services, usually because services are not covered by your policy, because you did not follow the plan's rules (such as getting preauthorization for a service from the plan) or because the insurer's medical officers do not consider the treatment medically necessary for you based on their knowledge, policies, or current accepted standards of prescribing. See "Letters of Medical Necessity" to understand how doctors can respond to a denial of coverage.

Disabled. A person who is crippled, injured, or incapacitated is generally considered to be disabled. However, in insurance, it may be defined according to the terms of your contract, with no specific universal understanding. The customer should call the health insurance provider to get a specific definition of how that policy at the specific carrier defines "disabled."

Discount Plan. This is not insurance but rather a prearranged discount pricing agreement between medical service providers and the health plan administrators.

Effective Date. The date your insurance is set to actually begin. You are not covered until the policy's effective date. If you have been uninsured for a period of time before your new health insurance policy is issued, effective dates may vary for various underlying conditions. A customer may call customer service to learn about rolling effective dates for various conditions after a plan starts.

Employer Waiting Period. Found in an employer group health plan, this is the amount of time a new employee must wait, , before being eligible for health care coverage. This waiting period is managed by the employer. It is usually used to avoid hit-and-run behavior by a new employee, in which the employee files a large claim right after joining and then quickly leaves the company. It also helps to minimize paperwork for employers with high turnover of employees. Also see "Affiliation Period."

The Employment Retiree Income Security Act (ERISA). Passed in 1974, the legislation allowed employers to design their own coverage packages and refuse to cover things like in vitro fertilization or to satisfy state requirements for minimal mental health coverage.[2] The passage of ERISA had a destabilizing effect on the health care delivery system. As firms self-insured their employees, relatively healthy and higher-paid employees were withdrawn from the risk pools covered by private insurance companies. This left behind a smaller population of less healthy individuals and resulted in an increase in premiums, which made it more difficult for smaller employers to offer health insurance coverage to their employees.[3] "ERISA is a federal law that preempts state laws making employer-sponsored plans largely exempt from state benefit mandates and consumer protections ... The 130 million Americans enrolled in ERISA-protected plans cannot sue their insurance company or employer in state court if they have been denied coverage for a treatment or procedure ... [Health insurance companies] like ERISA ... [because] it allows insurers to thumb their noses at state laws designed to protect consumers against insurance company abuses."[4]

Exclusion. Medical services that are not covered by your insurance policy are considered excluded. Specific exclusions to your coverage may be provided by your health insurance provider by request from the customer service department. Not all exclusions are always listed in the summary statements that are distributed with your policy.

Exclusion Period. The amount of time a new health plan member must wait to get coverage for care related to a preexisting condition. The length of this type of waiting period can vary from one to eighteen months.

Explanation of Benefits (EOB). The insurance company's written explanation of a claim that generally shows the patient's financial obligation to a provider of services. It may also provide a summary of the amount paid by the policy and the usual and customary charges submitted by the claimant but not the actual amount paid or an explanation for the denial of a claim.

Fee for Service. Payment to doctors, hospitals, and other health care providers for each service they give a patient. The provider itemizes or invoices the insurance company for each billable product or activity performed. The opposite of fee for service is capitated payment for services provided.

Federal Employees Health Benefits (FEHB) Program. Health insurance benefits offered to employees of the federal government, including members of Congress. Like private employers, the government contracts with private insurance plans across the country to provide benefits to federal employees. The government, as the employer, subsidizes a portion of the premium of the plan the employee selects.

Fiduciary. A person to whom property or power is entrusted for the benefit of another, putting the other person's needs above any possible needs or conflict of interest of the provider of the trust.

Formulary. The list of drugs a health insurance plan will cover at some level under particular circumstances. There are often tiers within the formulary for drugs within a particular class for which the insurance company pays a specific price. Tier-one drugs have the lowest co-pay and are often generics. Tier-two drugs cost the patient more out of pocket because they may be branded or they may be more expensive therapeutic options for the health insurance company to procure from the drug company. There are usually tiers of "preferred drugs" within a particular class of therapy.

Guaranteed Issue. A consumer protection offered by some states and the federal governments that gives people the right to buy health insurance coverage regardless of age or health status.

Guaranteed Renewability. A consumer protection that gives people the right to keep their health insurance coverage regardless of age or health status but at a price the insurer determines. In order to keep a guaranteed renewable policy in effect, customers must always keep their premiums paid and up to date.

Group Insurance. A group health insurance policy is sold to cover a large number of people affiliated by a common risk group or employer. Everyone in the group gets the same coverage for the same price. The insurance company spreads the risk equally among the healthy and the sick in the group.

HIPAA (Health Insurance Portability and Accountability Act). HIPAA amended the Employee Retirement Income Security Act (ERISA) to provide new rights and protections for members of group health plans. HIPAA contains protections both for health coverage offered in connection with employment (group health plans) and for the availability of individual insurance policies sold by insurance companies to people who previously had group coverage.

HMO (Health Maintenance Organization). A type of managed care plan that generally covers only the care you get from doctors, hospitals, and other health care providers that are in the plan's network. HMO members generally must choose a primary care doctor who acts as the "gatekeeper," deciding when they can go to a specialist.

In-Network. Doctors, hospitals, and other health care providers that contract with a health plan to treat plan members. Policyholders usually pay a lower co-payment when using in-network providers because the providers have agreed to provide services at lower reimbursement.

Indemnify. Insurance is designed to guard or secure the policyholder against anticipated or unanticipated loss. It protects the policyholder for an unexpected expense incurred as the result of a loss, illness, or accident and compensates for damage or financial loss sustained.

Indemnity Health Plan. These are the fee-for-service types of plans that primarily existed before the rise of managed care plans like HMOs. In an indemnity plan, you pay a predetermined percentage of the cost of health care services, and the insurance company pays the other percentage. For example, you might pay 20 percent for services, and the insurance company pays 80 percent. Indemnity health plans, also called fee-for-service plans, give you the freedom to choose any health care provider.

Individual Insurance. A health insurance policy sold to an individual and not as part of a group. Individual insurance policies are generally regulated by the states, so rules vary widely across the country. Individual insurance policies are generally more expensive and less comprehensive than group policies.

Length of Stay (LOS). A term used by insurance companies, case managers, and/or employers to describe the amount of time an average individual may stay in a hospital or inpatient facility for hassle-free payment of the claim. If a claimant requires a longer stay, the physician may need to submit a letter of medical necessity to assist the facility in receiving an additional payment and to justify the charge.

Letter of Medical Necessity. When an insurance company questions the doctor's decision, the doctor may provide in writing a letter with supporting evidence from medically scientific and relevant journals, explaining why that medical direction is recommended. This is how the doctor may refute the health insurance company's decision not to pay for a product or procedure.

Lifetime Maximum Benefit. The maximum amount a health plan will pay in benefits to an insured individual during that individual's lifetime. The policyholder should know this figure before agreeing to the policy. Insurance is designed to protect you against financial disaster, and a cap, or maximum benefit, limits the completeness of that protection. This practice is illegal, except in certain circumstances, as a result of health care reform.

Limitations. A limit on the dollar amount of benefits paid out for a particular covered expense as disclosed on the certificate of insurance. Customers may contact their health insurance providers to request a copy of the limitations of their plans.

Limited Benefit. Maximum dollar benefits defined for various conditions.

Medicaid. A joint state and federal program that provides health care coverage to people with very low incomes who meet eligibility criteria, such as being a child, being pregnant, being a single parent, having a disability, or being sixty-five years of age or older, with very limited income.

Medicare. The federal government program that provides health care coverage to people sixty-five years of age or older and people under sixty-five who have a disability, no matter their income or state of residence. The vast majority of people with Medicare (about 75 percent) get their medical benefits directly from the government-administered public program. The rest have joined a private insurance company that contracts with the government to provide benefits to people with Medicare.

Medical Loss Ratio (MLR). "By jacking up premiums and shifting more and more cost to their policyholders, insurers are able to manipulate an obscure ratio that is especially important to their shareholders: MLR. It is telling that insurers consider the amount of money paid out in medical claims to be a loss. (Some companies now call it by other names, such as the 'benefit ratio,' which may sound more palatable.) When an insurer lowers its MLR, it is spending less on medical care and more on overhead ... If an insurer reports that its MLR was lower during the preceding quarter than the same quarter a year earlier, it means the company spent less on medical care— and therefore had more money left over to cover sales, marketing, underwriting, other administrative expenses, and most important, profits. This, in turn, pressures insurers to be vigilant in finding ways to cut their spending on medical care, and this vigilance has paid off: Since 1993, the average MLR in America has dropped from 95 percent to around 80 percent."[5]

Medical Underwriting. An insurance company practice that bases the premium and sometimes the benefits on an individual's own medical history. So the premium for people who are sick or who are likely to become sick (for example, people with diabetes) is higher than for people who are healthy.

"Must Issue" State. A state that mandate issue health insurance providers to an applicant regardless of underlying medical conditions, providers that may not decline an applicant that is willing to pay the premium charged for that policy in a "must issue" state.

Medically Necessary. Procedures, services, or equipment approved as necessary for the diagnosis and treatment of a medical condition. Every health insurance company has a staff of physicians that evaluates the standard approaches to care for every illness or disorder. Thus, what one company determines to be medically necessary may not be the same thing as what another company decides.

Network. A group of doctors, hospitals, and other health care providers contracted to provide services to an insurance company's customers for less than their usual fees. Provider networks can cover a large geographic market or a wide range of health care services. Insured individuals typically pay per usage for using a network provider.

Out-of-Network. Doctors, hospitals, and other health care providers that did not agree to the terms of payment your insurance plan's network offered are referred to as "out-of-network." If you get services from an out-of-network provider, it usually means that you will have to pay for more or all of the costs for the services you received.

Out-of-Pocket Costs. Health care costs that you must pay because your insurer does not cover them. Similar to cost sharing.

Out-of-Pocket Maximum. A predetermined limit on the amount of money you must pay of your own money each year on medical costs before your insurance company will pay 100 percent of your health care expenses.

PCP (Primary Care Physician). The doctor that manages your care and refers you to specialty care when needed is referred to as a PCP or may also be called a "gatekeeper." A managed care plan like an HMO generally requires you to have a PCP. If you don't consult your PCP before seeing a specialist, your managed care plan will likely not cover your care. PCPs can be general or family practitioners, internists, pediatricians (for children), or gynecologists (for women). Plans without gatekeepers generally indicate NG in the plan title.

POS (Point-of-Service) Option. A type of HMO that provides plan members partial coverage for certain services they receive outside the managed care plan network of providers. You can choose providers within the health care network or outside. Costs per visit are lower, and the level of coverage is higher with in-network services. You may need to get referrals from your primary care provider to seek treatment from specialists. You may pay deductibles and higher coinsurance rates with out-of-network providers.

PPO (Preferred Provider Organization). A PPO is a type of managed care plan that should partially cover the care from out-of-network providers. However, to get full coverage, you must use network providers. Enrollees generally pay a higher annual premium for this flexibility and a higher contribution at the time of service.

Preadmission Certification. Approval by an insurance company representative for a patient to be admitted to a hospital or inpatient facility, granted prior to the admittance. Preadmission certification may be obtained by either an individual or a physician. For many plans, if you do not get preadmission certification, the plan will not pay for the services provided.

Preauthorization. Also called "preapproval," it is an approval that a managed care plan member must ask for from the plan or primary care doctor before getting certain medical services. In some plans, if you do not get preauthorization, the plan will not pay for the care received.

Preexisting Condition. A medical condition or disease you have or had prior to joining the health plan. The exact definition of a preexisting condition and how long a plan can look back in your medical history to find a preexisting condition varies by the type of plan. For employer group plans, regulated by federal law, the health plan can only look back six months prior to joining the plan and can only exclude coverage for your condition for up to eighteen months. The amount of time the plan can exclude coverage depends on how long you were without coverage for that condition prior to joining the plan. For individual and small group plans, regulated by state law, the rules vary widely by state. Some states allow the plan to look back years into your medical history and exclude coverage for that condition forever; other states limit the health plans to looking back six months and exclude coverage for no more than six months. Check back for updaters as health care reform evolves.

Prescription Tiered Pricing. Tiers within the formulary for drugs within a particular class for which the insurance company pays a lower price, such as generic drugs, that have a corresponding lower co-payment. Tier-one drugs have the lowest co-pay and are often generics. Tier-two drugs have a higher co-pay and may be branded or more expensive therapeutic options within a particular class of drugs.

Premium. The amount of money a consumer and/or an employer pays monthly to an insurer for health care coverage.

Preemption. Health insurance is governed by the laws of each individual state. A few federal laws also govern health insurance. When state and federal laws conflict, federal law overrides or preempts state law.

Private Insurance. Insurance coverage provided by a nongovernment entity, where the private company takes on the risk of insuring its members. Private insurance companies can be not-for-profit but are most frequently for-profit businesses.

Public Plan. Insurance coverage provided directly by the government, where the government takes on the risk of insuring its members. It is always not-for-profit.

Qualifying Event. There are federally recognized times during a plan year for which customers may amend their policies. These events may result in a change of premium. The events include but may not be limited to a death of a covered person, the birth or adoption of a dependent child, a marriage, or change of employment status of the covered individuals. Changes usually need to be made in writing to the carrier within thirty days of the date of the event in order to secure coverage effective at the date of the event.

Reasonable and Customary Fees. The average fee charged by a particular type of health care provider within a geographic area. The term is often used by medical plans as the amount of money they will approve for a specific test or procedure. If the fees are higher than the approved amount, you may be responsible for paying the difference.

Referral. Authorization that managed care plans usually require for services not provided by your primary care doctor. Policyholders in "gated networks" must get a referral from their primary care doctors in order to see a specialist or get certain exams. A "gatekeeper" is responsible for generating the referral.

Rider. A modification made to a certificate of insurance regarding the clauses and provisions of a policy (usually adding or excluding coverage).

Risk. Insurance is based on risk. When you get an insurance policy, the insurance company is taking on some of your risk. The relative risk is based upon the chance of loss, the degree of probability of loss, or the amount of possible loss due to an accident or illness. Where costs are known, predictable, and manageable, there is no need for insurance.

Risk-Based Rating. Setting premiums based on an individual's likely health care needs. For example, somebody who already has diabetes or has a family history of diabetes would be charged more than somebody with no health problems. The difference in premiums would reflect the difference in expected health care costs for each policyholder. Risk-based rating is the opposite of community rating.

Risk Pooling. Risk pooling groups many people together to share (or spread) the costs (or risk) generated by a small number of people. The number of people covered makes up the pool of people in the plan.

The State Children's Health Insurance Program (SCHIP). SCHIP is a joint state and federal government program that provides health care coverage to families with children. The program was designed to cover uninsured children in families with incomes that are low but too high to qualify for Medicaid. SCHIP benefits are provided through private insurance companies that contract with the state.

Service Area. The geographical area within which a health plan provides medical services to its members. In an HMO, it is the area where your network of doctors and hospitals are located.

Single-Payer System. A government-based health care system that handles all insurance plans and claims, as opposed to the multipayer system used in the United States. Sometimes the terms "universal health insurance" and "single-payer system" are interchanged as equivalents, but they are really entirely different concepts.

Specialist. A physician who specializes in treating only a certain part of the body or a certain condition. For instance, a cardiologist only treats people with heart problems.

State Continuation Coverage. A law enacted in most states that extends COBRA-like rights to people who work for companies that have fewer than twenty employees. In some states, these laws apply to fully insured group coverage purchased by larger employers as well. However, there is little uniformity between each of the states with regard to qualifying events, duration, covered benefits, and the cost of state continuation coverage. Each state defines different qualifying events that trigger the right to continue group coverage. Depending on the state, these qualifying events are not necessarily the same as those under COBRA. Also, most states require people to have been covered under their group plans for a minimum period (such as three months) in order to be eligible for state continuation coverage. By contrast, COBRA only requires a person to have been covered under the group health plan on the day before the qualifying event.

Underwriter. An underwriter's job is to make sure that the insurance charges just the right amount for the coverage it provides. They figure how much risk you represent, how much coverage the company can offer you, and how much that coverage should cost. Every insurance application passes through an underwriting process, and every application is evaluated by a professional whose opinion is going to determine how much you pay for insurance. Based on the condition of your health—or even a mistake on your application—an underwriter could decide to deny your application entirely. Applying for insurance leaves a record. If you get denied coverage, it will show up in that record. Once you've been denied coverage at one company, other companies are more likely to deny you too.

Universal. Policies available to all applicants regardless of health history or other personal or demographic considerations.

Usual, Customary, and Reasonable (UCR) Rates or Covered Expenses. An amount customarily charged for services and supplies which are medically necessary, recommended by a doctor, or required for treatment. This amount varies from insurance company to insurance company and may not actually represent the contracted amount paid to the product or service provider.

Voluntary Benefits. Benefits that are paid 100 percent by the employee. The employer offers the benefits to the employee but is not willing to a pay a portion of the premium. The rate of the plan is lower than could be achieved if the employee tried to purchase the same plan outside of the group. These benefits are usually deducted from your payroll check, either pretax or after tax, and the premiums are subsequently remitted to the carrier by the employer.

Waiting Period. The period of time specified in a health insurance policy that must pass before an applicant is eligible to be enrolled in a company-sponsored health insurance policy.

Endnotes

Foreword

[1] http://www.bls.gov/news.release/cesan.nr0.htm.

[2] http://www.creditloan.com/infographics/how-the-average-consumer-spends-their-paycheck/.

[3] "Health Benefit Costs in Private Industry," Bureau of Labor Statistics, Daily Report, June 11, 2009. http://stats.bls.gov/opub/ted/2009/jun/wk2/art04.htm.

[4] "Hospital Component of MEPSnet," AHRQ, http://www.meps.ahrq.gov/mepsyoub/data_stats/MEPSnetIC.jsp.

[5] "2008 Healthcare Cost and Utilization Project Nationwide Inpatient Sample," AHRQ.

[6] http://www.nfpa.org/assets/files/pdf/os.fireloss.pdf and American Hoyouing Survey for the United States: 2009, Series H150/09. U.S. Department of Transportation, National Highway Traffic Safety Administration; Federal Highway Administration http://www-nrd.nhtsa.dot.gov/Pubs/811402EE.pdf; auto insurance injury claims http://www.ircyoub.org/news/20080213.pdf.

[7] 2011 Milliman Medical Index: Healthcare Costs for American Families Doubles in Less than Nine Years. May 2011.

[8] "Health Insurance Industry Profits Surge Again: Fewer members, Skimpier Benefits, Lower Spending on Care Add up For Investors While Consumers Suffer," Health Care for America Now, May 2010, http://hcfan.3cdn.net/d605c2281191ac1f04_kam6bn3ga.pdf.

[9] ibid.

Chapter 1

[1] "Recent Challenges to the Use of 'Usual, Customary and Reasonable' Medical Provider Charge Data for Price Reimbursement Implications for Payors and Providers," Janov, Locke Lord Bissell & Liddl, American Health Lawyers Association, 2008, http://www.lockelord.com/files/News/347b7836-0e69-4059-ae76-03ae268243a1/Presentation/NewsAttachment/c89438e7-58af-47d1-8f7c-16699b7ba0f0/HLWarticle2.pdf.

[2] Potter, p. 121.

Chapter 2

[1] ibid.

[2] ibid.

[3] Paul vs. Virginia, 75 U.S. 168, 19 L. Ed. (357) 1868.

[4] Mayhall, Val III, http:// www.insuranceregulatorylaw.com/2011/05/brief-chronicle-of-insurance-regulation.html A Brief Chronicle of Insurance Regulation in the United States, Part 1: From De Facto Judicial Regulation to South-Eastern Underwriters Ass', Insurance Regulatory Law.

[5] The McCarren-Ferguson Act, 15 U.S.C. 1011–1015.

[6] Mayhall, Val III. A Brief Chronicle of Insurance Regulation in the United States, Part ii: From McCarran-Ferguson to Dodd-Frank, Insurance Regulatory Law

[7] Kwon, W. Jean (2007) Uniformity and Efficiency in Insurance Regulation: Consolidation and Outsourcing of Regulatory Activities at the State level, Networks Financial Institute, Indiana

[8] Clayton M. Christensen, *The Innovator's Prescription: A Disruptive Solution for Health Care* (New York: McGraw-Hill, 2009), 224.

[9] ibid.

[10] Isadore S. Falk, et al., *The Cost of Medical Care* (Chicago: University of Chicago Press, 1933).

[11] Stabilization Act of 1942, Title 50, Appendix "War and National Defense" (1942).

[12] Christensen, 226.

[13] Maggie Mahar, *Money-Driven Medicine: The Real Reason Health Care Costs So Much* (New York: Harper Collins, 2006).

[14] J. Newhouse, *Handbook of Health Economics*, 646–706.

[15] Christensen, 227.

[16] Christopher J. Conover and Ilse R. Wiechers, "Cost of Health Services Regulation Working Paper Series: HMO Act of 1973," Duke University, April 2006.

[17] Ziming Liu, *Paper to Digital: Documents in the Information Age* (Westport, CT: Greenwood Publishing Group, 2008), 78.

[18] ibid.

[19] "Guaranteed Availability Under Title XXVII of the Public Health Service Act – Applicability of Group Participation Rules," Department of Health and Human Services Memorandum, Insurance Standard Bulletin Series,.November 2000,. http://www.cms.gov/HealthInsReformforConsume/downloads/HIPAA-00-05.pdf.

[20] http://www.badfaithinsurance.org/reference/HL/0118a.htm.

[21] ibid.

[22] "13 Things Your Health Insurer Doesn't Want You to Know," Center for Health Insurance Claims Advocacy, http://www.claims-advocacy.org/13_things_your_health_insurer_do.htm.

[23] ibid.

Chapter 3

[1] Janov, Locke Lord Bissell & Liddl, 2008.

[2] http://www.newchoicehealth.com/Directory/Procedure/28/Digital%20Mammography%20-%20Both%20Breasts%20(Mammogram).

[3] Kaiser Family Foundation, March 2009

[4] Milch, et al., "Voluntary Electronic Reporting of Medical Errors and Adverse Events," *Journal of General Internal Medicine* 21, no. 2 (February 2006): 165–170.

[5] Regina Herzlinger, *Who Killed Health Care?: America's $2 Trillion Medical Problem—and the Consumer-Driven Cure* (New York: McGraw-Hill, 2007), 227–246.

[6] Kaiser Family Foundation, "Trends in Health Care Costs and Spending," March 2009.

[7] Paul B. Ginsburg, "Can Hospitals and Physicians Shift the Effects of Cuts in Medicare Reimbursement to Private Payers?" *Health Affairs*, Web Exclusive (October 8, 2003), W3-472 to W3-479.

[8] M. A. Morrisey, "Hospital Cost Shifting, a Continuing Debate," EBRI Issue Brief no. 180 (Washington: Employee Benefit Research Institute, 1996).

[9] J. A. Rizzo and D. A. Blumenthal, "Is the Target-Income Hypothesis an Economic Heresy?" *Medical Care Research and Review* 53, no.3 (1996):274–287.

[10] http://content.healthaffairs.org/content/early/2003/10/08/hlthaff.w3.472.full.pdf.

[11] Wendell Potter, *Deadly Spin: An Insurance Company Insider Speaks Out on How Corporate PR is Killing Health Care and Deceiving Americans* (New York: Bloomsbury Press, 2010), 121–124.

[12] "Health Care in America Survey," ABC News / Kaiser Family Foundation / USA Today, October 17, 2006, http://www.kff.org/kaiserpolls/upload/7572.pdf.

[13] Stephanie Kelton, "An Introduction to the Health Care Crisis in America: How Did We Get Here?" Special Series on Healthcare, Center for Full Employment and Price Stability, 2007, http://www.cfeps.org/health/chapters/html/ch1.htm#_ftn21.

[14] Ida Hellander,,"A Review of Data on the U.S. Health Sector," *International Journal of Health Services*, Vol. 36, No. 4 (2006): 787–802.

[15] "The Uninsured: A Primer, Key Facts About Americans without Health Insurance," November 10, 2004, Henry J. Kaiser Family Foundation and Health Research Educational Trust, http://www.kff.org.

[16] Kelton,.

[17] ibid.

[18] Paul B. Ginsburg and Len M. Nichols, "The Health Care Cost-Coverage Conundrum: The Care We Want vs. The Care We Can Afford," *Health System Change*, Annual Essay (2002–03) , Center for Studying Health System Change, http://www.hschange. com/CONTENT/616.

[19] C. Borger, "Health Spending Projections Through 2015: Change Horizon," Health Affairs Web Exclusive, February 2006, W61: 22.

[20] Kelton.

[21] ibid.

[22] "Health Insurance Cost," National Coalition on Health Care, 2007, http://www.nchc.org/facts/cost/shtml.

[23] David U. Himmelstein, Elizabeth Warren, Deborah Thorne, and Steffie Woolhandler,, "Market Watch: Illness and Injury as Contributors to Bankruptcy," *Health Affairs*, February 2, 2005, http://content.healthaffairs.org/cgi/content/full/hlthaff.w5.63/DC1.

[24] National Coalition on Health Care, "Health Insurance Cost."

[25] Sara R. Collins, Karen Davis, Michelle Doty, and Alice Ho, "Wages, Health Benefits, and Workers' Health," *The Commonwealth Fund*, Issue Brief, October 6, 2004.

[26] Robert W. Seifert, "Home Sick: How Medical Debt Undermines Housing Security." November 2005 (Boston, MA: The Access Project).

[27] Kelton,.

Chapter 4

[1] Wendell Potter, **Deadly Spin**, pp. 144 - 145

[2] "Administrative Expenses of Health Plans, prepared for Blue Cross Blue Shield in 2009," Douglas B. Sherlock, http://www.bcbs.com/issues/uninsured/Sherlock-Report-FINAL.pdf.

[3] Kaiser Family Foundation calculations using NHE data from Centers for Medicare and Medicaid Services, Agency for Healthcare Research and Quality, Medical Expenditure Panel Survey (MEPS), 2006.

[4] Herzlinger, 105.

[5] ibid.

[6] ibid.

[7], "End Health Care Discrimination: Give Health a Chance," Georgia Public Policy Foundation, 2003, http://www.gppf.org/article.asp?RT=9&p=pub/HealthCare/Consumer-DrivenHealthCare/simple%20care.htm.

[8] Devon M. Herrick and John C. Goodman, "The Market for Medical Care: Why You Don't Know the Price; Why You Don't Know about Quality; And What Can Be Done About It," National Center for Policy Analysis; March 12, 2007.

Chapter 5

[1] Kaiser Family Foundation calculations using NHE data from Centers for Medicare and Medicaid Services, Agency for Healthcare Research and Quality, Medical Expenditure Panel Survey (MEPS), 2006.

[2] http://www.ncrponline.org/PDFs/Thomson_Reuters_White_Paper_on_Healthcare_Waste.pdf.

[3] ibid.

[4] "Administrative Simplification for Medical Group Practices," Medical Group Management Association, June 2005.

[5] "The Price of Excess: Identifying Waste in Healthcare Spending," http://www.pwc.com/healthindustries.

[6] http://www.ncrponline.org/PDFs/Thomson_Reuters_White_Paper_on_Healthcare _Waste.pdf.

[7] http://www.huffingtonpost.com/wendellpotter/insuranceindustryflack_b_864126.html.

[8] David E. Williams, "MinuteClinics and retail healthcare's tipping point," MedCity News, August 3, 2010, http://www.medcitynews.com/2010/08/minuteclinics-and-the-healthcare-consumers-tipping-point/.

[9] http://www.wejonesmd.com/Pages/Gen/overcharged.html.

[10] "Obama's Push for Healthcare Reform and Other Health News," US News and World Report, http://health.usnews.com/health-news/articles/2009/02/24/health-buzz-obamas-push-for-healthcare-reform-and-other-health-news/comments.

Chapter 6

[1] http://www.bls.gov/news.release/cesan.nr0.htm.

[2] http://www.creditloan.com/infographics/how-the-average-consumer-spends-their-paycheck/.

[3] "Health Benefit Costs in Private Industry," Bureau of Labor Statistics, Daily Report, June 11, 2009,. http://stats.bls.gov/opub/ted/2009/jun/wk2/art04.htm.

[4] "Hospital Component of MEPSnet," AHRQ, http://www.meps.ahrq.gov/mepsyoub/data_stats/MEPSnetIC.jsp.

[5] "2008 Healthcare Cost and Utilization Project Nationwide Inpatient Sample," AHRQ.

[6] http://www.nfpa.org/assets/files/pdf/os.fireloss.pdf and American Hoyouing Survey for the United States: 2009, Series H150/09. U.S. Department of Transportation, National Highway Traffic Safety Administration; Federal Highway Administration http://www-nrd.nhtsa.dot.gov/Pubs/811402EE.pdf; auto insurance injury claims http://www.ircyoub.com/news/20080213.pdf.

[7] 2011 Milliman Medical Index: Healthcare Costs for American Families Doubles in Less than Nine Years. May 2011.

[8] Potter, 118.

[9] "Reality Check: AHIP's 'Study' Hard to Take Seriously," White House Blog, October 12, 2009, http://www.whitehouse.gov/blog/Reality-Check-AHIPs-Study-Hard-to-Take-Seriously.

Chapter 7

[1] "Health Insurance Industry Profits Surge Again: Fewer members, Skimpier Benefits, Lower Spending on Care Add up For Investors While Consumers Suffer," Health Care for America Now, May 2010, http://hcfan.3cdn.net/d605c2281191ac1f04_kam6bn3ga.pdf.

[2] ibid.

[3] Potter, 106.

Chapter 10

[1] "Prescription Drug Trends," Kaiser Family Foundation, May 2010, http://www.kff.org/rxdrugs/upload/3057-08.pdf.

[2] ibid.

[3] Tod Marks, ,"Consumer Reports Study: Comparison Shopping for Prescription Drugs Saves Big Bucks," September 2008.

Chapter 13

[1] Herzlinger, 145.

[2] http://www.irs.gov/pub/irs-drop/rp-10-22.pdf.

[3] http://www.irs.gov/pub/irs-drop/rp-10-22.pdf.

[4] http://www.irs.gov/pub/irs-pdf/p502.pdf.

Glossary

[1] Adapted from thefreedictionary.com, dictionary.com, and http://www.insurancecompanyrules.org/pages/glossary/.

Endnotes

[2] David Blumenthal,. "Employer-Sponsored Health Insurance in the United States—Origins and Implications," *The New England Journal of Medicine*, July 6, 2006, 82–88, http://www.nejm.org.
[3] Kelton.
[4] Potter, 178.
[5] Potter, 121.

About the Author

Katherine Woodfield, a twenty-year veteran of medical and health sales, received her MBA from Penn State University. A veteran employee of such great companies as GlaxoWellcome, Pharmacia, and Sanofi-Aventis, Ms. Woodfield was trained to assist in patient reimbursement from the perspective of the pharmaceutical industry. Ms. Woodfield, a two-time cancer survivor, used her personal experience and augmented her knowledge during her late husband's journey into medical expenses to launch her career into brokering health insurance. Ms. Woodfield's goal when evaluating health insurance options for her clients is to "protect her clients against financial disaster, while buffering them from high premiums." She sees herself as an educator, a guide, or an instructor, teaching her clients the simple methods they may employ to reduce health insurance premiums, protect their families, and eliminate financial risk.

Ms. Woodfield graduated from Princeton High School and received her bachelor's degree from Pine Manor College in Chestnut Hill, Massachusetts. She went on to receive her MBA from Penn State with a focus on marketing. She spent the next fifteen years, through the Clinton administration, working for major US pharmaceutical companies and learning how the pharmaceutical industry worked with, through, and for its end consumers, the everyday patient. During those years, she was exposed to the explosive growth of the HMO industry and moved from a primary care environment into an oncology- and research-based focus. As marketing regulations tightened, drug formularies were born, and patients began paying for medical goods and services they had never paid out of pocket for in the past, she worked with various entities to help patients gain access to vital medical therapies.

A survivor of her own personal medical battles, Ms. Woodfield took her career in a new direction after the death of her children's father. After experiencing a great loss, knowing the feeling of uselessness and helplessness where nothing can be done to change the course of events, Ms. Woodfield took all her new knowledge and power and set out on a quest to help the average person understand the health insurance plan options from which they are being asked to choose. One group at a time, Ms. Woodfield has reduced premiums, empowered employees with understanding, and expanded coverage to people who had never had coverage before.